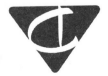

Others Are Saying

"Communication skills and techniques are Drebinger's trademark. He presents safety and health subjects in a magical way that makes audiences hang on every word. His communication techniques make it easy to recognize unsafe conditions and acts in the work place."

Jerry P. Ray, CSP

"John Drebinger is a great communicator. I've been to many of his seminars and used him several times in our company. I always come away with many notes and new ideas. Now he's done an outstanding job putting his ideas in book form. This is a must read for all safety professionals!"

Bob Johnson, Safety and Training Manager
Granite Construction Inc.

"John Drebinger is a master communicator!! His wit, passion, and ability to combine safety concepts with entertainment are unique and groundbreaking in the safety profession. Read this book and use these skills!!"

Hal Taylor, CSP

"John Drebinger truly masters the art of safety communication in his new book. I've successfully integrated several of John's techniques into my own motivational safety and keynote presentations. The feedback has been fantastic. It's like adding magic to technical information. Don't wait to buy this book."

Bruce S. Wilkinson, CSP
Professional Speaker / Consultant
Workplace Consultants Inc.

MASTERING SAFETY COMMUNICATION

Communication Skills For A Safe, Productive, and
Profitable Workplace

John Warner Drebinger Jr., C.Ht., CSP
Certified Speaking Professional

Revised First Edition

Wulamoc Publishing, Galt, California

MASTERING SAFETY COMMUNICATION

Communication Skills For A Safe, Productive and Profitable Workplace

By John Warner Drebinger Jr., C.Ht.

Published by:
Wulamoc Publishing
Post Office Box 1406
Galt, CA 95632-1406 U.S.A.

Copyright © 1997, 1998, 2002
by John W. Drebinger Jr.
First Printing 1997, Second Printing 1998, Seventh Printing 2002
Printed in the United States of America
Cover design by Ad Graphics, Tulsa, Oklahoma
Phone: (800) 368 6196

Library of Congress Cataloging-in-Publication Data
Drebinger, John W., Jr.
MASTERING SAFETY COMMUNICATION: Communication Skills
For A Safe, Productive and Profitable Workplace
by John Warner Drebinger Jr. 1st ed.
Includes bibliographical references.
Library of Congress Catalog Number: 97-90019
ISBN 1-890296-00-7 (pbk.)

Order Information

To order additional copies of this book or to receive information about other products and services by John W. Drebinger Jr.

Contact:
John Drebinger Presentations
13541 Christensen Rd., Suite 200
Galt, CA 95632

Phone:
(800) 588-9419
(209) 745-9419

Visit Our Website:

http://www.drebinger.com

E-Mail:

john@drebinger.com

Be sure to sign up for :

"John Drebinger's Dynamic Safety Meetings Report"
Weekly Electronic Newsletter
Available **Free** Online

Also By John W. Drebinger Jr.

"Mastering Safety Communication"
Audio tape of book by the same title, unabridged.

"Dynamic Safety Meetings Institute Home Study Course"
Audio CD's of entire three day institute.

"John's Magic Kit"
Magic kit and instructional video.

"Creativity and Safety Training Techniques"
Audio tape.

"Safety Summary Cards"
Summary of Key Points from John's Presentations.

All available by calling:
John Drebinger Presentations
1-800-588-9419
or 1-209-745-9419

Or Online
www.drebinger.com

Also,

"John Drebinger's Dynamic Safety Meetings Report"
Weekly Electronic Newsletter
Available **Free** Online
Signup at: www.drebinger.com

Warning - Disclaimer

This book is designed to provide information on communication skills. It is sold with the understanding that the publisher and author are not engaged in rendering legal, accounting, or other professional services. Also, the author, while an expert in communicating safety messages, holds the National Speakers Association's highest earned credential, Certified Speaking Professional, CSP. He is not a Certified Safety Professional, also coincidently using the initials CSP. If legal or other expert assistance is required, the services of a competent professional should be sought.

It is not the purpose of this book to reprint all the information that is otherwise available to the author and/or publisher, but to complement, amplify, and supplement other texts. You are urged to read all the available material, learn as much as possible about communication, and to tailor the information to your individual needs. For more information, see the many references in the resource section.

Safety is a serious subject and if you aren't sure about technical issues you should consult someone who is qualified to give you the right information.

Every effort has been made to make this book as complete and as accurate as possible. However, there **may be mistakes** both typographical and in content. Therefore, this text should be used only as a general guide and not as the ultimate source of safety communication information. Furthermore, this book contains information on communication skills only up to the printing date.

The purpose of this book is to educate and entertain. The author and Wulamoc Publishing shall have neither liability nor responsibility to any person or entity with respect to any loss or damage caused, or alleged to be caused, directly or indirectly by the information contained in this book.

If you do not wish to be bound by the above, you may return this book to the publisher for a full refund.

Acknowledgments

One of the special privileges of writing a book is that you get to publicly thank people who have had a profound effect on your life. This is where I get to thank some of the people who have helped me on my journey. For the average reader, these people may be unknown, but I wish you had the opportunity to enjoy the pleasure of knowing them as I have over the years.

First, my Mom and Dad, Bernadette and John Drebinger, for giving me life and always being there to help and guide me. My wonderful wife, Karen, who has stood beside me for the past 31 years of marriage and always been there when I needed her. My children, Jessica and Johnny, for being the best kids I could have ever hoped for.

Denis Waitley, who was the first personal development speaker I ever heard, for teaching me to always say a simple thank you and to never pre-qualify to the negative. Anthony Robbins, a dear friend, and one of the greatest communicators in history. He taught me how to use my Personal Power to grow and stretch and many of the techniques I share with others. Dr. Tad James, Dr. A.M. Krasner and Dr. Richard Neves who taught me hypnosis and Neuro-Linguistic Programming.

Pacific Gas and Electric personnel for calling on me years ago to do a magic presentation at one of their safety kickoffs that introduced me to the field of safety.

Diane Weiss, who works day and night to market my presentations all across this country. Her dedication to this effort allows me to continue to compile and create new material and applications of the skills I have learned over the years. She takes the best care of my clients and me.

Loren Slocum for showing me how to inspire others to raise their own standards.

Cliff Dochterman and Rick King, two of my fellow Rotarians, whom I watched and modeled as outstanding speakers.

The Boy Scouts of America where I learned to teach, train, and entertain.

Bruce Wilkinson, for introducing me to the National Speakers Association, which has helped my career profoundly. Shep Hyken, who provided a model and advice on how to best transition from magician to an outstanding speaker. Larry Winget, who taught me, "If you believe in what you have to say and care about your audience you really need a book. To have something good to say and not offer it in every imaginable format is a disservice to those who need it and want it."

I also am grateful to God for the direction He has given me in life and to the outstanding model teacher, Jesus, who in addition to giving his life for me, also showed me and the world how to teach and communicate most effectively. Pastors of the churches I have attended over the years, Fred Doty, Robert Blacka, Luther Tolo, Vern Holmes, Charlie Knorr, Scott Minke, Tim Stevenson, Darrel Deuel, Richard Eddy, and Robert Salge. Their teachings have planted many seeds, which have developed into the ideas I share with others today. To Steve and Karen Oeffling who are outstanding models of service and ministry.

Alan Rosen, a friend as dear and close as a brother, whom I can always laugh with and count on.

Sarah Victory, my speech coach, who knows how to take what I do and make it better.

Sandie Gilbert, my editor, who on many occasions worked late into the night in order to make me appear to be literate.

My good friend, Dr. E. Scott Geller, whose research reminds us why and how people behave the way they do.

Special thanks to Jim Wolfe, Bobby Johnson, and Ken Schriner for checking out the cover photos for safety issues. My peer reviewers, Bob Johnson, Matthew Stasior, (Dr. Energy) and Hal Taylor, CSP.

And thank you to all those safety professionals who work day in and day out to create a safe workplace.

Dedication

There are places along the pathway of life where you come in contact with someone who has a profound effect on the path you take. My pathway to serving those in the field of safety was opened by a wonderful gentleman who was willing to give me a chance and opened the door so I could grow and expand into a new area of service. Every year in Anaheim, California the state's largest safety convention takes place. This event, sponsored by the Greater Los Angeles Chapter of the National Safety Council, draws several thousand safety professionals and people from businesses who have been assigned the responsibility of safety for their company or their department. This diverse group has the potential to impact the behaviors of thousands of employees throughout the Southwest.

My introduction to this event came when Joe Kaplan, President of the Greater Los Angeles Chapter National Safety Council called my office. Joe had heard I was doing a series of employee motivational presentations for Pacific Gas and Electric. Apparently comments about the effectiveness of my training techniques were quite positive. Joe contacted me and asked me if I would be willing to do a two hour seminar for the attendees of the convention. I was thrilled and apprehensive at the same time. Up until then I had only spoken to employees and had not trained members of the safety profession.

I wrote a special presentation entitled "Communication Skills for the Safety Professional." Thanks to Joe's confidence and encouragement the presentation was a huge success and from there my career jumped to a national level. Had he not invited me to stretch and raise my standards I would have continued speaking only to employees to motivate them to work safely.

As a result of my accepting his offer I have now been able to multiply my effectiveness by sharing my training skills with others. He also had the vision to invite me to share some of my rather unique methods with his clients.

Since then he has brought me on as a member of the Faculty of the Greater Los Angeles Area Chapter of the National Safety Council. I consider this a great privilege and an honor. Joe is the most dedicated safety professional I have ever met. He truly gets great joy knowing that his efforts are protecting people he will never meet. I am sure there are many people in this country today that owe their safe behavior to Joe and the safety professionals he has led and inspired over the years. I can only hope to have a fraction of the impact he has had and will continue to have for years to come.

Thank you, Joe, for your inspiration, love, and confidence. I will never be able to repay you for your kindness but I will strive to do so by serving others as you have done for so many years.

Table Of Contents

Chapter Contents Preview

Introduction

You have an exciting opportunity to affect the lives of numerous people, many of whom you will never know. Among these are the employees you train, their children, families, friends, and the public with which they come into contact. It is unlikely you will ever see the ripple effect caused by a person who performs a job safely or acts safely in their daily life. One way of looking at how far reaching your influence is would be to imagine an unsafe act, which results in an injury or death. The employee is affected, their family is affected by the loss of income and the change or absence of the person they love, and the community is affected where they lived and worked. On a more positive note imagine the effect you would have on the future history of our world if the safety information you impart saves the life of a person, who gives birth to a future inventor or world leader. It is no less profound to a child who has the joy of his parents coming home safely because of the work you have done. The impact of your success may never be known by you.

During the past several years it has been my privilege to train many employees to work and live safely. Whenever possible, I sit in on other safety presentations and take notes. It is obvious that there are many outstanding individuals dedicated to saving lives who are loaded with great knowledge, but many are looking for more effective ways to communicate their message to others. To achieve my goal of having a positive impact on others in the safety profession, I have developed a seminar entitled, "Mastering Communication". This seminar teaches skills that any safety professional, manager, or employee can use to make their communication of safety concepts effective. This book contains much of the material covered in my one-day seminar, plus some additional information. I hope these ideas will be useful to you in your efforts to make this a safer world.

Since the first printing of this book in 1997, I have had the privilege of speaking for hundreds of companies across this country. While doing so I have learned so much more than could fit into one book or one single day. Because of this, I have developed a three-day seminar called the Dynamic Safety Meetings Institute. It uses this book as the prerequisite course and goes way beyond. Many of the safety professionals and communication experts I have worked with over the past several years have shared with me some of their best secrets and I have combined them with what I have learned while speaking to thousands of people. One thing I know is that I will continue to learn and I encourage you to do the same. I hope this book is a step along your journey to becoming the best communicator you can be. When you have finished this book, please consider joining me for further learning. I look forward to talking with you in the future and I am always available by email at, john@drebinger.com .

I invite you to approach the material in this book with what Denis Waitley calls, "open-minded skepticism." Open-minded enough to try it out and see if it works for you and skeptical enough, that if it doesn't fit your situation, to set it aside and look for something else.

This book is written for people who are passionate and committed to achieving a safe workplace and making a difference in the lives of employees and their families as well as future generations. You are a very important and influential person who is dedicated to serving others and always searching for effective ways to create a safe workplace. You are joining over 35,000 people who have read this book as of this printing. I hope you find the tools in it as useful as they have. Enjoy using these techniques and skills to make a difference in our world.

"If you can't annoy somebody, there's little point in writing."

-Kingsley Amis

Chapter 1

How To Use This Book

"Committing your thoughts to print creates a void in your mind which your creative spirit will fill with new ideas"
                                        -- John W. Drebinger Jr.

"Writing down your thoughts is like planting them in fertile soil."

- John W. Drebinger Jr.

Write Down Your Ideas

While reading a book written by a friend of mine, I found that as I read it I was coming up with all sorts of ideas I could use in my speaking career. I happened to be on a short commuter flight and didn't have my laptop computer out for taking notes. I also had no paper with me. I know from experience that if I think of a good idea and fail to write it down I will forget it. I took out my pen and proceeded to fill the space on the inside of the front and back covers as well as several partially blank pages with my notes. Once home I transferred these ideas to the journal in my computer. Had I not gone to the effort of writing them down, several ideas included in this book would have been lost. You may have experienced talking with someone when you thought of a great idea and sure enough later in the day you struggled with, "What was that idea that occurred to me earlier?" This can be costly as sometimes you may never remember the idea.

This experience generated the placement of an idea section in the back of this book in order to facilitate your remembering and taking action on the ideas at a later date. If you record them on a separate piece of paper I recommend you also write them into the book as they will always be where you may refer to them. Not to mention, the book becomes more valuable to you each time you pick it up to add more thoughts. You won't want to lend your notated copy to a friend so you will just have to buy another one from us. All kidding aside, with the notes recorded, you always know where to find them.

Questions Can Be Your Compass

The direction your thinking takes is quite often directed by whatever question you are attempting to answer at the moment. Questions may give either positive or negative direction to your life. Questions contain a bias which will effect the answers you get. The questions we ask direct the results we achieve so it is important to design the questions you ask yourself to insure a positive result. For example, if you ask, "Why can't I come up with any good ideas for safety meetings?" You will end up with a list like:

- I'm not creative.
- I've tried everything.
- I'm just not good at this sort of thing.

If you ask, "What new ideas could I come up with for my next safety meeting?," you will get a better list. On occasion you might get stuck and not be able to come up with an answer. The basic technique in dealing with this is to respond with the following question or a slight variation thereof.

"I know I don't know _____, but if I did what would it (or they) be."

For example, consider the above question, What new ideas will I come up with for my next safety meeting? If you were stuck you ask yourself, "I know I can't come up with any new ideas for safety meetings but if I could what would they be?" If you need further assistance with this, check Chapter Eight, "Creative Ideas".

If you are aware that questions direct and help how you think, it would be a good idea to make effective use of them when writing and reading a book. When I began to write this book I had to ask myself, "What is my purpose in writing this book?" Some of the answers I discovered are:

- To serve others by sharing some of the communication skills I have learned and currently use.

- To have a book for the many people who have asked for one.
- To provide a written resource for those who attend my seminars.
- To have an example of my work for those considering using my services.
- To enable managers, trainers and safety professionals to become effective communicators resulting in fewer workplace accidents.
- To make a difference and contribute.

The next question that directed my writing was, "What is the desired outcome the book should achieve for the reader?"

- To give you, the reader, skills which will give you the ability to change the behaviors of the people with whom you communicate.
- To give safety professionals strategies, which will allow them to create a safe workplace by motivating employees to work safely.
- To allow you to become proficient in skills which will enable you to improve your effectiveness in motivating employees to be safe.

Reading This Book Effectively

For years educators and reading comprehension experts have said that students should read the review questions at the end of each chapter before reading the chapter in order to get the most out of it. If this is really effective, and I believe it is, then why not put the questions at the front of each chapter? So in order to increase comprehension I have taken two steps you might find helpful. First, prior to the "Introduction" there is a section titled, "Chapter Contents Preview" (page 17). Its purpose is to alert your mind to the topics covered in the entire book and in each chapter. If you haven't read this already please take a moment and do so now. The second step is a set of questions at the beginning of each chapter. Read these prior to reading that chapter. The following question is repeated with each chapter because it is designed to help you come up with some of your own ideas. What ideas in this chapter can I use to improve the safe behavior of myself and those with whom I work? I know you don't know which ideas you could use but if you could what would they be?

I will let you in on a secret as you read some of these questions. They will have words in them that have not been defined in the context of this subject. This is done intentionally, as it will cause your mind to be slightly confused and evoke a state of searching for the answers.

As you read and discover answers to the above question quickly write them down in the back of the book. When you are done reading review your ideas and then write down actions you can take immediately which will start the ball rolling.

Chapter 2

Communication Philosophy

"The effectiveness of communication is gauged by the results."
— John W. Drebinger Jr.

Questions To Enhance Your Reading

1. What ideas in this chapter can I use to improve the safe behavior of myself and those with whom I work?

2. What must I do to improve my skills as a communicator?

3. What are three ways I affect company profits?

4. How can I do my job and have fun at the same time?

There Are No Rules! Well Maybe One!

Throughout this book I will mention that you must do "whatever it takes" to make your safety message heard. It is important to understand the context of that comment. I believe that people have the right to come to work without fear of being harassed or mistreated. Any sexual, racial or inappropriate references or stories are not part of what we do. There are an infinite number of ways to get a point across in an interesting or unique fashion and still be appropriate in the workplace. A good rule of thumb is that if you are unsure something may be inappropriate assume it is and leave it out. The doubt you are feeling just might be a hint from your unconscious mind that someone could be hurt by that particular comment. It is always better to err on the side of caution. My reputation as a safety speaker has been based upon the evaluation by others that my material is always appropriate and takes no chance of embarrassing the corporate clients I represent.

Given that basic premise I then approach communication with a great deal of flexibility which will be discussed later. There are no rules other than being appropriate in the workplace. It is important to explore and build on your skills and the best way to do this is to try new and different things all the time.

Taking Personal Responsibility - A Key To Being Safe
Responsibility must be taken in many forms to assure a safe workplace. In order to be effective in communicating safety concepts each one of us must take responsibility for our own safety. As safety professionals and managers we must also take responsibility for the safety of those people in our jurisdiction. You and I must also take responsibility for the effectiveness of our communication. The effectiveness of communication is best judged by the results you get. You must do whatever it takes to be effective as a safety communicator, trainer, manager, or fellow employee.

This can be a disturbing concept for some people. After all, how can you really be responsible for the way people react to your communication? However it is critical for you to take that position because once you do you can search for solutions which will create results. Staying in a powerless state immobilizes your mind and removes any incentive to solve the communication problems you encounter.

Even if you have trouble believing that you must take personal responsibility I encourage you to "act as if" it were true and your brain will do the rest.

In Order To Make A Difference, You Must Believe You Can Make A Difference
Since I began speaking to employees about safety I have always taken the opportunity to interview the safety professionals who worked at the company. I discovered that there are two types of safety professionals, those who believe they make a difference and those who believe they do not. It doesn't seem to matter whether upper level management supports them or whether they feel the employees are committed to safety. Those who believe they make a difference have an attitude, which allows them to be more effective. It appears that the effective safety people are the ones who focus on their successes and look to create more.

Not too long ago I met safety executives in the construction industry at a meeting in Seattle and observed individuals who loved their profession, were committed to the outcomes they were responsible for and did not whine about what they could not do. After observing these professionals I decided that these are the type of people I want to serve as my primary target market. They are people who are committed to improving what they do and they seek out solutions instead of wallowing in their problems.

As a result of watching these professionals I decided to create a special focus for my company. In order to meet the needs of clients it is important for me to be able to clearly communicate to others what service I provide. In fact I developed an answer to the question, "What do you do?" following that meeting. "I work with companies that are committed to safety. I help them improve the effectiveness of their communication skills. "

"The mere belief that you can do something begins the process that makes it happen."
                    -- John W. Drebinger Jr.

Changing Who We Are Is How We Move To The Next Level Of Excellence

In order to move forward and improve, we must change who we are. People who never move forward and improve often find themselves saying, "If I did that I wouldn't be me." That is absolutely right. The person you are today is different from the person you were when you left elementary school. What you have learned through your life experiences has brought you to where you are today. The secret to success is to be committed to constantly learning so that the person you are becoming is better and more effective every day.

Whenever you review your materials or notes and are making changes, you should notice that what you are doing today is much better than what you did even six months ago. I am constantly astonished, when I watch video tapes and listen to the audio tapes of my presentations, how much I have improved. You may even have the privilege of having others comment on how much you have improved since they last saw you. Oftentimes they even apologize for the comment but it is a wonderful compliment for you if you are committed to constant improvement. It is a sign that you have grown beyond what was once your best. As long as you continue to grow and improve, you will be better able to serve those for whom you are responsible.

This book will give you some ideas that you have never used before and, as you use them, the person you are will change and improve as you make them a part of the way you communicate with others.

If you are truly committed to creating a safe workplace, you must always raise your own standards. No matter how good you become, you must enjoy your success and then challenge yourself to achieve yet a higher level.

Quite often when faced with change we find ourselves saying, "If it ain't broke, don't fix it." That may be true and what you are doing might be very effective but in order to progress you must change what it is you are doing or you will become stagnant. It doesn't make sense that the same behaviors or techniques we are using today will achieve better or different results tomorrow. You must always strive to find new and interesting ways to improve.

"The only thing scarier than change is being left behind."

                                            -- Jim Connery.

Create For Yourself The Role Of Someone Who Helps Supervisors Achieve A Safe Workplace

What areas of your responsibility as a foreman or manager would you be willing to turn over to someone not in your chain of command or directly responsible for your production and profitability? I imagine most people would answer, none, to this idea yet, why are they willing to allow the company safety professionals to be responsible for their workers' safety instead of taking personal responsibility and using the safety pro as a resource to assist in achieving the goals of production and profitability in a safe fashion.

As a safety professional you can multiply your effectiveness when you work with those in supervisory positions. You may empower them to use their authority to insure their employees are behaving safely, after all they are the ones who are in contact with the employees on a daily basis. Imagine your effectiveness if, instead of teaching employees to wear safety glasses, you teach their supervisors, who then take responsibility to see that their employees use them. This is vital because the employee is accountable to his or her supervisor and not necessarily to the safety professional.

Reinforce In Your Mind And Others That You Are Effective

When you have been successful motivating an employee to work safely write down how you inspired that behavior. When a person in your area of responsibility does well record their action. This will create a journal of successes. Your journal may be a record of how you make a difference in the lives of others. Positive comments from employees about your presentations and stories of employees whose behavior has changed should be included. Keep track of instances when foremen or supervisors have successfully used your ideas. A journal such as this is a resource for strengthening how you and others feel about the job you are doing. When something works write it down, whenever you receive positive comments from someone ask them to write a memo including the comments, then enter it in your journal.

Share this journal and its contents with your supervisors and managers. Quite often we don't get the recognition or budget we deserve because no one realizes the results of our work. How can they recognize the value you add to the company unless you share the differences you make? When someone in production increases their output it is obvious, but the effect we have is not as visible. Accident records alone do not necessarily have the impact on management that dollars saved will.

At the end of each month review what you have written in your journal. Every year read the comments you have recorded over the past few years and you will discover that you have improved indeed.

Earlier in this book the value of questions was discussed. Your journal is a great place to write the questions that will lead to the solutions you need to achieve. After you have written the question allow your mind to formulate the answer over time. When you discover an answer record it in your journal. If it isn't the exact resolution to the problem it might lead you to find the best solution.

Safety Professionals Affect Company Profits

If your company has a sales force paid on commission, figure out how much you saved last year. You may either show lower workers compensation costs or specific savings that safe behavior created. How much would you have been paid if you received the same commission as the salesmen for that increase in company profit?

Learning, Communicating and Entertaining

Steve Allen once said, "People will pay more to be entertained than to be educated." Walt Disney realized that through an entertaining medium you could teach and inform. I learned to entertain while growing up as a member of the Boy Scouts. I now believe that what I learned to do was to communicate effectively. Stories and skits were fun and often taught something at the same time. Much of what we were taught was through games or stories. As I learned to share entertaining and meaningful stories I realized the extent to which people enjoy listening to them and therefore discovered the value of entertainment as a tool to carry a message effectively. While humor and entertainment are great tools they are best used when they are relevant to the purpose or desired result. For the best results use jokes and stories that pertain to your message.

"Good teaching is one-fourth preparation and three-fourths theater."

-- Gail Godwin

Have Fun!

Be playful – with yourself and your audience. If you are having fun it is also likely your audience is. What an impact that would have on safety professionals or managers. Thomas Edison said he never worked a day in his life, to him it was all fun. Billy Graham, the well known evangelist, says that he wants to be remembered because he was fun to live with. These effective people discovered that when you are having fun doing what you love you are going to be effective.

"Work is either fun or drudgery. It depends on your attitude. I like fun."

-- Colleen C. Barrett

Do You Enjoy Results Or Just The Struggle?

Have you ever heard the saying, "Arguing with a safety professional is like wrestling with a pig in the mud. Pretty soon you realize you're not getting anywhere and the pig likes it." While this is a funny line it may just illustrate why some of us do not achieve results. Unfortunately, many safety professionals like to wrestle with people and not really gain results. We must be the type of professional that doesn't get stuck in his or her own mud but achieves results. Our mission is to help people be safe not to argue with them or their supervisors. If you ever find yourself stuck in the mud be reminded of your real goal and make a difference.

Believe In Yourself And What You Do

Ultimately, the key to your success is what you are willing to believe you are capable of doing. You must re-evaluate this on a regular basis. I can assure you upon being asked several years ago if I would ever write a book I would have said I doubt it. Since I continually stretch and work to improve I am now writing to share what I have been taught. I hope you enjoy the same growth as you use these techniques in service to others.

Chapter 3

Representational Systems

"To effectively communicate, we must realize that we are all different in the way we perceive the world and use this understanding as a guide to our communication with others."

-- Anthony Robbins

Questions To Enhance Your Reading

1. What is my primary representational system?

2. What ideas in this chapter can I use to improve the safe behavior of myself and those with whom I work?

3. What does my brain use to record and describe the world?

4. How could I motivate people by using sensory words?

What Are Representational Systems?

You observe the world using your five senses: eyes-(visual); hearing-(auditory); touch-(kinesthetic); taste-(gustatory); and smell-(olfactory). The information you gather about the world around you is recorded into your memory. The way your brain uses these inputs is the way you represent the world around you. The three primary systems are visual, auditory and kinesthetic.

In the field of Neuro-linguistic Programming there is a saying, "The map is not the territory." This is one way of saying whatever you notice or record about your world is unique to you. The meaning you give an event may be different than the next person's, therefore your view and representation of things is going to be unique. This explains why several people witnessing the same event from almost exact locations will describe it in many different ways. Their representation of the event is only a model, not the real event, and therefore is slightly different than what actually happened. Now you can see why sometimes your communication to others seems to be ineffective. Your model and theirs may be radically different and this confuses the message you are conveying. Even our closest friends and relatives have a different viewpoint than we do. Another way of looking at it is expressed by the saying, "Walk a mile in my shoes." This implies that if you saw things the way I did, you would understand me. On the positive side, being aware of this allows us to adapt and use alternative methods of communicating concepts to someone until we arrive at the result for which we are looking.

"Primary Representational System"

One representational system is stronger for every person so it is used and developed more. It becomes their primary representational system. It is the one you pay the most attention to and the one you use the most to describe, internally and externally, the world around you. It is important, as you begin to study these communication techniques, to realize that you represent the world around you using all senses but you favor one over the others.

A person using the visual mode as their primary representational system will notice visual things most frequently and use visual references in remembering things and describing them to others. I am a visual person and I therefore, tend to notice that which I see more than what I hear, feel, smell, or taste. I will use visual words to describe concepts or events to others. I am not sure I have what is called a photographic memory but I can create a visual picture of past events and use it to remember who you are and where you were sitting in one of my training sessions.

As a visual person sitting by a waterfall at Yosemite National Park I might remember the colors, the rapidly moving water flowing downstream. An auditory person might recall the sound of the water roaring as it hits the rocks below. A kinesthetic person might remember the cool mist hitting their face. The exact place and time but three distinct experiences.

Remember, you create an internal representation of the world around you. You tend to represent things in either a visual, auditory or kinesthetic mode. The primary modality you use is your primary representational system.

How To Use Representational Systems Effectively

When you are speaking to an individual you should strive to use their primary representational system. If you want me to understand and accept what you are going to tell me use the phrase, "John, you can *see* what a great idea this is." On the other hand selling the same idea to an auditory person you might say, "This sounds like a great idea, doesn't it?" The kinesthetic person would respond well to, "This just feels like the right idea." Now, I can hear some of you saying, "Wait, this is much too complicated. I don't want to have to figure out what system someone is using." In that case you can balance your speech by using all three representational systems so your message will be understood by everyone. The following story is an example of such usage.

Several years ago I was in Florida when a tragic traffic accident occurred. While *watching* the evening news I *heard* reports of the accident. A gasoline tanker truck was approaching an intersection which was just on the other side of some railroad tracks. Upon driving onto the tracks the truck got caught in a traffic gridlock. The driver placed his fate into the hands of the driver in front of him instead of taking personal responsibility and making sure there was plenty of room for him to pull forward and clear the tracks. You guessed it, at that moment a train arrives. Unable to stop in time the train hit the gas truck and the resulting explosion and fire cost seventeen people their lives.

As you know most people killed in fires die from smoke inhalation and never experience the *pain* of *burning*, but not these seventeen people. It was summer in Florida so most people are driving in a closed air conditioned car to avoid the *heat* and *humidity*. Imagine the horror as they *saw* the fuel cover their car and ignite. *Feeling* the *heat* radiate through their windshield and *watching* any passenger, possibly their child in the front seat,

seared in the heat. *Hearing* the *sound* of the
explosion in that slow motion world that occurs
whenever things seem to go wrong that they even
heard the *screams* of their children and themselves.
Feeling the intense *heat* of their last breath inhaling
the super-*heated* air *searing* their lungs.

For those lucky enough to escape death
imagine what they *saw*, *feeling* the radiating *heat* as
you *watched* people trapped in their cars knowing
there was no way you could help them. Only able to
listen to the *screams* and *watch* the inferno. You can
even imagine the *smell* and *taste* of smoke and *fumes*
in the air. All this because some truck driver placed
his safety in the hands of someone else and did not
take personal responsibility.

Analysis of Sensory Words Used In Story
In the preceding story I italicized the words that are
sensory based. If you read it again you can pick them out.
Below I have listed them by category.

Visual Words
burning, saw, watch, watched, watching,

Auditory Words
heard (2), hearing, listen, screams (2), sound.

Kinesthetic Words
feeling (3), heat (4), heated, humidity, pain, seared, searing

When I tell this story during my safety presentation I
can watch and tell which people are kinesthetic as I watch
them respond to the kinesthetic words. The auditory
people react as I use words describing or representing the
event in sounds. The visual members of my audience react
as they actually create a picture in their minds of the event.
The kinesthetic and auditory people are creating their own
feeling or auditory representation of the event internally as

well. By the way did you notice I even snuck a gustatory (taste) and olfactory (smell) reference into the story.

As you learn to use a variety of these systems you will find you are getting better results when you talk and write information for others. For example when discussing the importance of using safety glasses, an item obviously tied to vision, you can employ all three representational systems.

You can see the impact that losing your sight would have on your career, your family and your life. Imagine what it feels like to have to rely on only your other four senses to experience the world around you. Reaching out to touch that which you could once see would be a tough experience. It just doesn't sound like a good idea to take a chance with your eyesight. It's important to hear that voice inside reminding you to put those glasses on before you need them.

You can read through the above story and make note of the three representational systems used. If you can spot them in the story above you have what it takes to use them in your own communication.

Examples of Representational System Words

Visual:
Burning, dimness, film, focus, gaze, glance, glimpse, hazy, illustrate, look, obscure, perceive, perspective, picture, pretty, saw, see, stare, survey, viewpoint, vision, watch.

Auditory:
Amplify, call, chatter, cry, groan, harmony, hear, heard, listen, loud, moan, music, noisy, scream, silent, sound, talk, tell, told, tune, voice, whine.

Kinesthetic:
Concrete, cutting, feel, feeling, firm, grasp, grope, handle, hard, heat, heated, humidity, hurt, pain, push, relaxed, seared, searing, shiver, smooth, soft, stir, swell, tension, throw, tight, touch, tremble, warm.

Which Is Your Primary Representational System?

An exercise you might find enlightening is to tape record one of your training sessions or a conversation with a friend (be sure to let them know you are recording). After recording the conversation, listen to it and determine which is your primary representational system. Knowing this, you can make it a point to include in your communication with others the other two representational systems in order to reach more people effectively. As with any skill, at first you have to concentrate on using all three but over time you will do it naturally when you speak to groups. Remember, when speaking to an individual you may use their primary system if you know it or can figure it out. If not, cover all three modes and you will increase your effectiveness.

Chapter 4

Rapport Skills

"Employees don't care about what you know about them, they care about how much you care about them."
                              -- Harvey Mackay

Questions To Enhance Your Reading

1. What ideas in this chapter can I use to improve the safe behavior of myself and those with whom I work?

2. What could I do that would cause someone to instantly feel like they had known me for years?

3. How can I change my communication style to become more effective at gaining rapport with my team?

4. What are five areas to match to gain rapport?

The Magic Of Rapport

When you have rapport with someone you feel you have a sense of commonality. When you are in a state of rapport with someone their unconscious mind accepts suggestions uncritically.

"Rapport is the ability to enter someone else's world, to make him feel that you understand him, that you have a strong common bond."
"It is the essence of successful communication."
- Anthony Robbins

Have you ever seen or met someone for the first time and immediately said to yourself, "I really like this person," or, "I don't like this person." This phenomenon of establishing instant rapport or having a gut feeling about someone is caused by how we observe the physiology of people. According to a UCLA study which investigated how congruent people were in their communication, 55% of your congruency in communication is displayed in your physiology, 38% in the tonality of your voice and only 7% in the words you use. If you have learned to gain rapport with someone simply by asking them questions and finding out what you have in common you have limited yourself. Since 55% of our communication with others is a result of our physiology we should concentrate our efforts in that area to develop commonality or rapport with people.

You may never have much in common with someone based solely upon conversation. By adding the use of physiology for building rapport then you have a possibility of gaining a greater level of rapport with someone.

Matching and Mirroring

A technique you can use to establish "instant rapport" without studying every move or posture in a book on body language is something called, "matching and mirroring." People tend to like or feel comfortable with people they perceive to be the same as they are. When you assume the posture, facial expression, blinking, breathing, and gesture patterns of the person you are with, their unconscious mind notices the similarities and feels comfortable with you or establishes "rapport." Using this technique will send them the message that you are someone they can feel comfortable with and will earn for you their respect. Obviously, the use of matching and mirroring physiology gives you a huge advantage, due to the role physiology plays in your communication.

You may have said to yourself about someone, "There is something about that person I just don't like but I don't know what it is." It could be as simple as your communication physiology and theirs do not match. Fortunately, this is easy to overcome using the technique of matching and mirroring. When you are matching their physiology you are eliminating barriers to your communication.

What Matching and Mirroring Is Not!

It should be pointed out that matching and mirroring is not the same as mimicking someone. The difference between a mimicking child and the process of matching and mirroring is that the child makes sure that their copying is noticed and oftentimes they even echo the words you are saying. Matching and mirroring is a very subtle skill. If you approach this with an open-minded willingness to experiment you will discover how effective this skill is, and that no one will consciously notice what you are doing.

More Detail On How To Match and Mirror

The process of matching and mirroring is to first observe the person you wish to match and mirror. Watch the posture with which they are standing or sitting. Look at their breathing and their facial expressions. When they are talking, notice how they gesture. As you are observing them listen to the types of words they use and their tonality. Begin by casually and naturally matching their posture and then their breathing. If they change position don't move instantly to the new posture but wait and shift moments later. When it is your turn to talk begin what you have to say by using the same words and or phrases they have just spoken. When you gesture use the types of gestures they use. This is such a subliminal communication method it has profound effects on achieving agreement.

Rules: "Look To Talk" And "Look To Listen"

When you talk with someone you have developed a pattern of how you like to listen and speak. Some people look directly at you when they talk and it is important to notice this trait if you want to effectively match and mirror them. If they have this "look to talk" rule and you look away or are doing something else as you talk to then they are not going to be as comfortable with you and therefore less open to your message. If you are talking to someone who prefers to look away or around as they talk you will distract them and create barriers to your communication if you look them straight in the eye when you talk to them. They may wonder why you are staring at their forehead. Be aware of their look to listen rule also. Some people look directly at you as they listen and when you are listening to them it is important to look while they are speaking or they are going to think you are not listening. Once again the opposite style is important. If they look away when they listen you must copy that behavior if you want to enhance your effectiveness.

When Not To Use Matching And Mirroring

For our purpose as safety communicators there are only a few situations where it would be unwise to use matching and mirroring. If you are dealing with some one who is in a state of depression, mad at the world, or mad at you it might not be useful to match and mirror them. Also, with today's concern over sexual harassment if you felt someone was receiving the message that you were attracted to them and you did not want to convey that idea you could focus on breaking rapport by not matching them at all.

Five Things To Match In Getting Rapport

1. Match the **representational system** they are using.
   Are they in a Visual, Auditory or Kinesthetic mode?
2. Match the **physiological state** they are in.
   What posture, gestures, facial expressions including blinking and breathing rate are they using?
3. Match the **voice** of the person.
   What is the pitch, speed and volume of their voice?
4. Match the **level of detail** they are using.
   Are they speaking in terms of general subjects, big chunks of information or going into great detail to explain specific bits of information? For example, if you ask me how my day was and I answer by telling you about everyone I met and talked with I would be dealing in great detail or small chunks of information. However if I answer, "It was a busy day. I accomplished a great deal.", you would know I use large chunks of information.

5. Match the **words** they are using. Can you use some of the actual words they are using in their conversation when you respond to them? Does the level of language they are using employ simple words or complex words? This works very well when you use the words they use when they like something. Such as, cool, excellent, great, awesome, nice, fantastic, etc.

Cross Over Mirroring

There are times when it is impossible or inappropriate to match the posture of another person. I am unable to cross my legs with the same flexibility as a lighter person, so I will move to a similar posture or ignore that one feature, if necessary. If a man and a woman were talking and she was wearing a skirt, there would probably be some ways the man might sit that would be inappropriate for the woman to match. The key is to use your own common sense and match what you can that is appropriate. Cross over mirroring is best described by example. If someone were tapping their foot and you couldn't tap your foot, you could tap your hand on the table at the same pace. Milton Erickson, one of the people who was studied to develop these techniques, had to use cross over mirroring because he was unable to always use the same part of the body due to his physical limitations.

How Do You Know You Have Rapport?

When you have established a state of rapport there should be no resistance from the person with which you are communicating. If you are still encountering resistance, continue to match and mirror all the aspects of the other person you can. Sometimes it just takes a little longer. You may have to get them to change their physiology or their position. You can do this by having them change chairs, get up and walk somewhere or other creative ways of getting them to move. Another indication you have established rapport with someone is a feeling of familiarity. They might even say something like, "Don't I know you from somewhere?" One of my favorite indicators of having achieved a state of rapport with someone is that you change your physiology and they follow you. Now they will be much more open to suggestions from you.

How To Achieve Rapport With A Room Full Of People

Many safety professionals do training, give presentations and of course, conduct many safety meetings with a variety of people in the audience. Unfortunately, some people don't even want to attend the meeting. The rapport skills you have learned in this chapter can help you make contact with difficult individuals in the audience.

The next time you are at a meeting notice the postures people assume as they sit in chairs or at a table. You will probably discover that there are only a limited number of possible positions available. A good strategy for gaining rapport with a group is to match and mirror any leaders within the audience. These leaders may be the actual official leaders but oftentimes are co-workers that their fellow employees follow or admire. Next, focus on matching and mirroring anyone you notice is resistant to the ideas you are teaching. If someone is being difficult you can eliminate the difficulty by matching and mirroring them. Lastly, match and mirror over the course of your presentation all the remaining types of physiology that it is practical to match. This allows you to make a real connection with the maximum number of people.

Chapter 5

Motivation Of Yourself And Others

"Enthusiasm is the footprint left by passion!"

-- John W. Drebinger Jr.

Questions To Enhance Your Reading

1. What ideas in this chapter can I use to improve the safe behavior of myself and those with whom I work?

2. What choices could I give people that would motivate them to work safely?

3. How can I evaluate my work as a safety professional so I can improve my own view of my effectiveness?

4. How can I increase my level of expectation from others and myself?

Take Responsibility For Training Results
In order to be successful I must take full responsibility for the results of this book. If this book sits on a shelf unread, it is because I didn't make it compelling enough to be read. If those who read it do not make use of its methods it is my responsibility.

For me to do anything less than take responsibility for my work will result in less than my best. Too many trainers look at external factors and prepare themselves an excuse for why their trainees did not succeed. Excuses do not achieve results, responsibility does.

I know there are many factors working on the people you train. Their emotional state, their physical state, their likes or dislikes of the subject, their bosses' support or lack thereof. And on and on and on....

If these circumstances are viewed as situations beyond your control then you will not seek to develop a training which will end in results instead of excuses. When we take responsibility we become leaders striving to motivate others to act with behavior that results in safety.

In the field of hypnotherapy there is an approach which teaches us that if you can put the client "at cause" or in a position of responsibility for the condition or problem they are experiencing then they can be "at cause" for a cure or change of behavior. This approach is useful to you as a communicator for if you consider yourself "at cause" for the results of training then your brain will seek out solutions to create the desired and demanded results.

"Do not wait for leaders; do it alone, person to person."
-- Mother Teresa

Making Safety Communication Important To You
Therefore, it is critical to put a person "at cause" to achieve results. The therapeutic setting also teaches us as trainers another empowering belief, "The client can only achieve that which the therapist believes he or she can achieve." In other words the clients progress is limited by the therapist's beliefs and limitations. This is also true for us as trainers. If we do not believe we can transmit this information to someone, then I assure you we will not accomplish the desired result.

In order for you to effectively communicate safety information, whether informational or motivational, it is important to develop a simple, but successful strategy. The nation's best trainer, Anthony Robbins, teaches the following formula for success.

- First, you must be in a peak state.
- Second, you must tap into your passion.
- Third, you must resolve to accomplish what you want.
- Fourth, you must take massive, intelligent and consistent action.
- Fifth, you must study your results, make adaptations and continue on with your presentation.

If you expect to effectively motivate or sell others to use your techniques and adopt new behaviors, you must have a positive vision of the outcome you desire for yourself and your audience. In order to be at a peak level of effectiveness I tap into my passion and create an outcome that is so compelling that my brain will absolutely create a way to succeed.

The vision which drives me and creates my passion is to motivate people to realize that they must take personal responsibility for their own safety. I believe that if they act from this belief they will follow their company's safety procedures and take an active part in being safe on and off the job. If, as a safety professional, I can provoke people to make safety a priority in their lives, I will in fact save lives as a result of my work.

Too often I have followed other speakers at many of my corporate training situations where the presenter preceding me had a great deal of lifesaving information but the audience wasn't receiving their message. They had no passion, enthusiasm, energy and therefore no impact in what they had to teach.

How To Build Passion

I practice a technique which allows me to increase in my mind the importance of the subject matter I am about to present and therefore it has allowed me to tap into my passion which carries over into my presentation for my audience. Prior to my presentation I envision the overall effect I will have on my audience. When I am training a group of twenty-five people I picture them internalizing my ideas thus changing the way they behave and also acting as a model for those around them, their family, co-workers, and friends. I then focus on the fact that I have an effect on more than just the twenty-five people I am training. It multiplies and spreads out like the ripple in a glassy pond. I will in fact affect thousands of people.

Next, in my mind I look for evidence that I am actually "making a difference." I was reading the National

Safety Council's accident statistics for one year and it refers to the fact that last year there were fewer industrial deaths than the year before. I thought about that for a moment and I remembered a seminar I took several years ago from a man named David Smith. He pointed out that during the years he had been teaching water safety, water fatalities had dropped. He then said the reduction was due to his work. Now I don't know if that was really the reason or if he believed it was due to him but it taught me something valuable. Whether he really believes this or just acts as if it were true, it certainly will change how excited and passionate he will be about his next presentation. When you believe you are making a difference it comes across in your work. I personally believe David has had that level of impact because he is an excellent teacher and trainer of trainers.

As a result of what I learned from David when I read about last year's accident record I made the following conclusion. I had my best year speaking to employees and managers about safety last year so it must be due to me that the number of industrial deaths dropped. If I take credit for that, what idea does that generate in my brain? It makes what I'm doing more important to me. I don't care whether other people believe I had that level of impact, but if I believe it, I will be excellent in my communication with my audience. How is that going to affect the physiology I mentioned earlier? If I really believe that by talking to any group that hundreds of people are going to be safer, I will get much more excited about my presentations. It elevates it from just a talk to a group of disinterested people to something worthy of my time and theirs. This excitement translates into energy and enthusiasm in my body and my delivery.

"Never doubt that a small, group of thoughtful, committed citizens can change the world. Indeed, it is the only thing that ever has."

-- Margaret Mead

Making A Difference

I have found that there is much more enjoyment and purpose in life if you make a difference. I really get excited about that. You see I am concerned about the employees that work for you as well as their kids. The kids arrive home from school and see Mom or Dad come home, all because of those who have learned from me and have created a safe workplace by conveying the significance of safety to their employees. So my audience gets an enthusiastic presentation and I get a great deal of personal satisfaction. That is why I love to teach and train. My primary purpose is that I get to make a difference in people's lives and as a side benefit I get paid. The financial reward is really a by-product of my having an effect on so many people's lives.

If you think about your job and the effect it has on other people, I guarantee you will surpass your former performance. Your brain suddenly says, "This is important. I should really focus on this." When you start taking responsibility, many great things will begin to happen. First, by taking responsibility for your actions, you will also have the right to receive credit when they are successful. If you take credit for the good things that have happened, as in my example where I had a great year last year and they had a better safety record than ever before, then what is that going to do for your level of motivation? You will realize that you have a responsibility for making it happen again next year. Therefore, you can continue to improve your presentations and become more effective because you will want to have an increased impact next year.

"I discovered I always have choices and sometimes it's only a choice of attitude."

-- Judith M. Knowlton

Motivation Idea - Choice

Give people two choices and make them responsible for the consequences of their choice. If they choose to behave unsafely they must realize it is their choice to accept the consequences. Likewise, they benefit by behaving safely.

For example, my daughter was complaining to me that she didn't always appreciate it when she did not have complete use of her room because of other family members using her computer. While she is the primary user of her computer her brother, her mom and I will be using the computer occasionally. I gave her a choice, the computer could remain in her room with the interruptions or we could take the computer out and put it into her brother's bedroom and move him into her room on a bunk bed. That way no one would be inconvenienced when others need computer time. Obviously, she is going to choose to have the computer in her room. This made the disruptions to her lifestyle seem much more acceptable.

Employees have the choice to work safely or face certain consequences. It, then, becomes their choice what result they achieve. If they choose to follow the safety procedures the consequences are positive and if not the resulting consequences will have a negative impact on their life.

Some companies give their employees the choice to work safely or work for someone else. Clearly this is a company willing to do whatever it takes to get an employee to work safely.

"Safety" Their Viewpoint or Yours

It is important when trying to change the behavior of others to discover what motivates them. The Boy Scouts of America has used a technique, which illustrates my point. When training Cub Scout leaders the trainer asks the adult leaders to get on their knees. It is then pointed out that this is how an 8-year old boy sees the world around him. If you can ask yourself, "What motivates or excites those I am training?", you will discover the way to get your message across to them. Remember it isn't what motivates you that counts, it's what motivates them. Some ideas you might consider are: family, sports or income. It is important to let them know that the real beneficiary of any safety program is themselves.

Safety And Production

I have discovered that companies with an excellent safety record also have a superior production record. Several reasons for this are that employees perceive that management is sincerely concerned about them and they respond by increasing production. Managers who are aware of the importance of safety and are concerned about their employees are typically better managers. Reminding employees to work safely is a reminder to them to do the job right and we know if they do their job properly, they will do it more effectively. Decreased accidents lessen losses, which directly saves you money.

The Magic Of High Expectations

Quite often trainers make a fatal mistake by believing that teaching or learning safety is boring. This is tragic because people respond to your highest expectations. If you believe you can make safety interesting and that your audience wants to learn how to take charge of their own personal safety they will respond accordingly. If you approach safety as boring then your employees will also treat it as such. Take a moment and do whatever it takes to get yourself in a positive physiological and emotional state so you can do your very best for those you have the privilege to train.

Back in the late sixties Scientific American completed research concerning the effects of expectation on results of teaching. They observed three classrooms of students that had been tested and found to be as close to equal in intelligence and ability to learn as could be determined. They randomly divided each class into three groups. Teachers were informed that ten students in their class were expected to do above average for the year, another ten were expected to do average and the final ten names were expected to do below average. After one year they looked at the results and also reviewed the observations of teacher behavior during the year. They found that the students' end of the year grades matched the artificially predicted results. In checking the observation notes it had been discovered that the teacher spent a little extra effort with those who were expected to do well and less with the group expected to show below average results. The conclusion was that expectations had a major influence. Once again proving that expectations are critical in achieving outstanding results.

My own speaking experience bears this out. Many times I have had someone tell me before a presentation, "This is a tough group." I proceeded as I always do believing that my audience wants to hear what I have to say and that they are capable of understanding all I have to give them. In almost every case the person who warned me returns after my presentation and exclaims how they have never seen the group so cooperative, attentive and responsive. It is no surprise to me because I expect that level of response from all the groups to whom I make presentations.

Just recently prior to a presentation for mechanics of a metropolitan transit agency, my assistant overheard one mechanic say to a coworker, "A one hour meeting, no way, I'll be out of here in five minutes." He had the expectation of not staying and leaving for some made up excuse. I, on the other hand saw him as someone who wanted to work without getting injured and therefore he would want to hear all I had to offer and listen to what I had to say because I knew how good my presentation was. My expectation came true. When I was done (right at quitting time I might add) several people stayed afterwards to talk with me and no one left early.

Safety Is A Team Effort

Safety is one of those things that becomes easier and more effective when handled as a team. It is fascinating to me that when I look out for you and you look out for me it doesn't merely double our effectiveness it geometrically increases. This phenomenon is the result of my awareness increasing. In order for me to watch out for you I must pay closer attention to hazards and as a result I see hazards I might have missed before.

Have you ever noticed that when you teach someone a skill you have recently learned, you also improve. Safety has the same benefit to you when you teach it to someone else or when you expand your awareness of safety from beyond yourself to include the members of your team. While the beginning of safety awareness is to take personal responsibility for your own safety, the next step is very important. You can raise your own personal awareness to the level of excellence by taking responsibility for the safety of those around you. When you do this you automatically or unconsciously become more aware of potential hazards because your focus is sharpened. So even by doing an unselfish thing of being focused on someone else's safety you end up doing something which directly benefits you. You become safer.

It is important to point out that you are probably a member of several teams. Your team at work, your team called your family, your team of friends, and your team of those you know in any organizations in which you are active. When you expand your awareness to the point of watching out for the safety of all those teams your record is bound to improve dramatically.

Taking Responsibility For Others Safety

Too often we see a problem and what do we do? We determine it to be someone else's responsibility. We must take it personally. You see, ultimately we are the real beneficiaries of our own safe behavior. When you take personal responsibility for your own safety you achieve one level of safety awareness. In order to progress from where you are today to being outstanding at safety you must continually raise your own personal standards. I suggest a very effective way to raise our own personal standards resulting in greater safety for us is to take personal responsibility for the safety of those around you. The magic of this approach is that we change our focus from ourselves to others and this ironically increases our own personal awareness. Have you ever experienced a situation where you had to teach something to someone? Isn't it amazing that as you go about the process of teaching something you know to someone else a benefit is that you become better at it yourself. This exercise changes your focus and expands your safety awareness beyond yourself resulting in your own enhanced safety.

Motivation Of Safety Professionals

While teaching the "Communications Seminar" for the New Mexico ASSE, I discovered a new way to motivate Safety Professionals to use the new communication skills they have learned. I asked them if they felt uncomfortable using the matching and mirroring techniques. Many indicated yes and I responded by asking them if any of their employees have ever told them that wearing safety glasses, respirators, hard hats, etc. was uncomfortable. They nodded yes and I responded that we know that even though those things are uncomfortable to them that they must use them for their own safety. It is much more important to place safety before comfort. Also, we know that when someone uses a safety device consistently enough they become used to it and it is oftentimes not uncomfortable any more.

Using these new motivational communication skills, that I am advocating, is no different. They seem uncomfortable to you at first, but after a while you will find they become easy. We know as safety professionals that if the information we want to convey is important, it is oftentimes a matter of life or death that we effectively

communicate in a way that changes employee behavior.
Not using the most effective communication skills would be
as irresponsible as not using safety glasses or a hard hat in
a hazardous area. We owe it to those for whom we are
responsible.

There is an interesting analogy in the above. I
realized that it seemed similar that some safety
professionals feel uncomfortable using new ideas as
employees feel uncomfortable using personal protective
devices. When I made this analogy the physiological
response in the room was awesome. I watched as the
concept hit them right between the eyes. I knew I had
made an effective point that they felt at the depth of their
being. It is so exciting when this happens! The same will
happen for you as you employ these skills with practice.

I want you to know that just as the techniques that
you teach are uncomfortable to them so are the strategies I
have taught you. You must make use of them because you
know that they will increase your effectiveness with your
students and you can give them nothing less than your
best.

**"Aerodynamically the bumblebee shouldn't be able to fly
but the bumblebee doesn't know that so it goes on
flying anyway."**
                                                  -- Mary Kay Ash

Reinforcing Your Own Effective Self Image

If you want to be an effective communicator follow
these two simple steps. Step one is to act as if you are an
effective communicator! Step two is to build references to
reinforce your belief. Your beliefs about your own
effectiveness will profoundly affect your communication
results as a safety professional. Keep a notebook of
positive reviews of your meetings. Keep any letters which
compliment you on your effectiveness. Keep several blank
pages inside so you can record any comments people share
with you verbally but not in writing. The availability of

comments in a notebook to review for future presentations offers you a resource to reinforce your opinion of yourself as an effective communicator.

Build Strong Beliefs About Your Effectiveness

Whether you believe you are a master communicator or not does not just drop on you from above. You are the one who develops your own evaluation of all that you do in life. Most of us look outside of ourselves to develop our sense of self worth and this can be limiting. In order to build a strong self image you can decide from within what you want to achieve, act as if you have achieved it, and then focus on the evidence that supports it. What you believe about yourself is developed every day of your life. Evidence of your effectiveness is received by you from many sources. The more people tell you that you are an effective safety professional or an effective communicator, the more likely you are to develop that belief. It is also possible to let negative comments or focusing on negative events create the belief that you are ineffective. The belief you have depends on which inputs you decide are significant to you. Your belief is the sum total of the evidence you have collected. In order to be effective it is helpful to act as if you are already a master communicator. Since this has such an effect you need to adjust your evidence collecting mechanism to focus on the positive. This makes it increasingly possible to do a better and better job. I should point out that this is not just fooling yourself into complacency because you connect it with continually making an effort to improve yourself. Remember, what you focus on is what you will become so focus on the positive and continue to improve everything you do.

Feedback Forms

Give yourself the gift of encouragement. Use this tool as a strategy to help you improve a great deal. The key is to understand that a feedback form will improve you if it focuses on your positive rather than the negative side.

Every personal development expert I have read tells you to take what you do well and improve it, then the negative points will take care of themselves or will be insignificant. In my experience, I have observed that God has given each of us certain gifts or talents. When we focus on using them to our best ability we make a difference in people's lives. It only makes sense to use and improve your strengths rather than focusing on your shortcomings and never making the real impact you were meant to make. Included is a sample feedback form for your use. Some key points about the following sample are:

1. It only asks positive questions. To ask what someone didn't like or what they would have left out presupposes that there was something they should have disliked or wanted removed. The questions you ask control what your attendees focus on. If you ask someone a question that requires a positive response it leads them to look for the positive. It's not just so you will look good on a form, it is a way for them to realize you are going to always ask these questions and they will pay closer attention in order to have something to write about.

2. You ask them to write down their name. This allows you to do follow up. If you have twenty people in a meeting and you get back ten forms you have some work to do. It is important to go to anyone not turning in a form and get their answers. This trains them that you are going to insist on their feedback, once again forcing them to pay closer attention. If they know you are going to ask them what they liked they will find something. Plus, you gain a list of things they liked, which is what you will continue to include in the future.

3. The form has no numerical choices because we want them to write down specific items. They have to think more to answer questions instead of merely circling numbers.

Feedback Form

Thank you for your participation in today's meeting. Please take a moment to give me your comments so that I may improve my presentations in the future.

What did you enjoy about today's safety meeting?_____
_____
_____
_____

What was something new you learned today?
_____
_____
_____

What is something you can use that you learned today?
_____
_____
_____

What did I do well at today's meeting?_____
_____
_____
_____

Is there anything else you want to say?_____
_____
_____
_____

Name:_____
Date:_____

Doing Whatever It Takes

When employees do not change behavior they just have not yet been convinced. You have not been willing to do whatever it takes to get them to work safely. You may decide that you have to remove them from your company because you do not have time to finish the job but if you keep them, you must figure out a way to get them to work safely.

In the movie, "Apollo 13", Eugene Kranz, when faced with the probability that the astronauts might not make it home alive, responded with a phrase that should be the motto of all safety professionals.

"Failure is not an option."

-- Eugene Kranz

When we all adopt this philosophy as our motto we make a huge leap towards success. Our minds then realize that we must succeed and so begin to search for the solution. We then, open our minds to do whatever it takes to succeed.

Passion

If you aren't passionate about a topic the likelihood of your communicating it effectively is very dim. Only a consummate actor could overcome a lack of passion and I don't know many Oscar-winning safety professionals. The beauty of being passionate is that it overcomes most of our communication shortcomings. People will not notice your lack of polish or the fact that you have an irritating style, etc. The person who is passionate about a subject will be forgiven much and their message will be remembered for a lifetime.

I remember when my friend, Dr. E. Scott Geller, was making a presentation on research. He was concerned that the audience would find it boring since it wasn't something exciting. What I observed during his presentation was that they were engaged and involved and actively listening because he displayed passion. When Scott talks about research he glows with excitement and passion. He still included humor and entertaining stories, which gave it his personal touch and left us all wanting more.

Bruce Wilkinson has such energy and passion you sometimes think he is going to leap right off the stage into your lap. Bruce, Scott, and I all have a passion for helping people avoid injuries. You should see what happens when we get together and talk about safety. Sitting across from each other at lunch or dinner you can sense the passion and excitement. I am sure if you had a heart monitor attached to us you would see our heart rate rise as we shared how we could reach people more effectively.

Even when our paths don't cross as we speak around the country an occasional phone call can change my day. Sadly, safety reports focus on injuries but when we talk with our fellow safety team members we can discuss and focus on our successes. This is a great way to build passion.

I suggest you find some fellow safety people to help you grow and nurture your passion. When you have had a tough day it can be empowering to talk to someone you know is as passionate as you are about the field of safety. If you don't have associates like that at your place of employment seek them out at safety conventions or meetings. Share what works for you and ask what successes they have had. Sometimes, their passion will ignite yours and you are renewed and ready to make a real difference in the workplace.

Chapter 6

Inspirational Learning

"Training and education without follow up and enforcement is usually ineffective."
-- Bruce Wilkinson

Questions To Enhance Your Reading

1. What ideas in this chapter can I use to improve the safe behavior of myself and those with whom I work?

2. Are the people I work with or encounter learning positive or negative safety behavior from others?

3. Do I follow-up and enforce what I teach?

4. Who could I study to be a student of excellence?

A Positive Effect Of Copying behavior

During my seminars I use magic to illustrate ideas or concepts. One trick I use to show people how they learn just by watching other's behaviors is the Needle Through the Balloon Effect. The trick is to stick an eighteen inch needle through an inflated balloon without it popping. I invite a member of the audience to assist me. I ask them to hold the balloon and I tell them their assignment is to stick that needle through this balloon without breaking it. At this point the person always stops and usually gives me a strange look. I point out that the person froze and did not do anything except look at me as if I were crazy. They did not even begin to figure out how to do it and therefore went into a "stuck" state. If you don't believe something is possible, your mind won't even try to discover a solution. If you want to find out how to be successful at things, you must first know where you are going. If you do not envision or know your destination, you will never reach it. If you visualize a picture of what you want to accomplish and you believe it is possible then you move in that direction. You must envision something yourself in order to achieve it. For example in order to realize a safe lifestyle, you must believe you can live and work safely and see yourself in that role.

Remember, I told the person holding the balloon to be very careful they do not pop the balloon. They stopped at that point and did not continue because they did not believe it was possible for them to accomplish the task. I then take the balloon out of their hand and proceed to stick the needle into one end of the balloon. It doesn't pop and the person has a confused look on their face. I then continue through the balloon and out the other end near the knot in the balloon and pull the needle all the way through. I then stop, toss the balloon into the air and pop it with the sharp point of the needle while I explain that it is not a trick balloon. I point out that the person was slightly confused because they walked into this room with a belief that sharp objects and balloons did not coexist. The person had a lifetime of references to back up that belief but now in a brief moment they saw that belief being challenged and removed by the evidence they were witnessing with their own eyes.

Something significant happens at this point. First, they go into a state of confusion which now prepares their mind for learning. When we are confused we are desperately looking for answers to that which confuses us. It is useful as trainers and managers to realize that we can make use of this phenomenon. I do so in this case by asking the person to now complete on their own the task I gave them originally. The person instantly begins to go to work. I point out at this time the difference in their behavior. The first time they were stuck, but now they know it is possible to accomplish so their brain quickly analyzes the situation and comes up with a solution. Since they know it can be done, they are much more willing to try it. It is also interesting to note that with all the people I have done this they have all modeled my behavior and stuck the needle into the end of the balloon where the rubber is the thickest and then moved it out near the knot where the rubber is also thick. Without even announcing that I was going to teach this trick I have done so by being an example of how it could be accomplished.

Bonus Of Working For A Safety Conscious Company
One of the benefits of working for a company that places an emphasis on safety is that your actions become safer and as a result your children and the people around you see safer behavior in you at home causing them to act accordingly. Just as the person modeled my behavior without instruction, those around us unconsciously model our behavior. As safety professionals and managers we must be consistent. It creates the wrong model when you say one thing and act in a different way.

The person with the needle and the balloon was modeling my behavior and learned by watching me. I did not say to the person that I was going to teach them the needle through the balloon trick. Not once did I mention that. They performed what we call in Neuro-linguistic Programming a technique called modeling. They watched what I did, ascertained what my strategy was and then copied it. That allowed them to be successful. The person was unconsciously learning while I was doing it. They noticed that I placed the needle in the end of the balloon where it is the thickest. As soon as it was their turn to do it they turned the balloon that way and started because they knew that was the successful method to accomplish the task. They learned all that unconsciously. That is very important when it comes to safety because you have people watching you all the time. People you work with may have a different reaction time than you do and you may have much more experience than they have. This might allow you to get away with a shortcut for a longer time without a disaster however by demonstrating the wrong way to do something you set others up for accidents because of what they learn by watching you.

One Way People Learn, On The Job Training
Many companies have formal training programs for new employees where they teach the official company policy about procedures which they believe are important. We know from experience that in addition to the formal

training an informal training period begins as soon as they begin work. This informal training is not presented by a supervisor using a manual or training materials. It is accomplished by the employee who observes the behaviors of all the employees and management at a company.

A new employee will quickly ascertain whether the written policies of the company are followed or ignored. If management is certain that their employees follow policy, they are exposing themselves to massive trouble with new employees. When it comes to safety there is the possibility of having new and inexperienced employees being taught to work in an unsafe manner. Whenever management ignores unsafe behavior they are condoning unsafe actions and in a sense permitting it to be perceived as company policy.

Correcting Unsafe Behaviors Is A Must

As managers it is critical to realize that when unsafe behavior by employees is tolerated or ignored their co-workers will learn by watching them. A poor example will teach others and set the stage for accidents. That is why it is important for everyone to be committed to safety to make it work for the entire team.

There may be a hotshot who thinks they know everything, which by the way is the type of thinking which commonly precedes an accident resulting in injury. Therefore, if a precedent for correct standards is established and followed, people will unconsciously model the safe behavior and lead a safe life.

As your safety record continually improves you become an exemplary model to other people. You create the belief in other people's minds that it is possible to work safely.

During my presentations I often ask for someone who is athletic with whom I can have a contest. Invariably someone points to their friend sitting next to them. I then say, "I always like to pick someone who points to someone else. You see by pointing at your friend you have committed an unsafe act." The selected volunteer from the audience remarks, "But he pointed at me first." I respond, "That's right, it often happens that way when it comes to safe or unsafe behavior. Someone else does something wrong and nothing bad happens to them. We observe their behavior and decide to copy their actions ignoring the safe procedures we are supposed to follow. What happens next? We face the consequences of the unsafe act." I use this interaction to illustrate that just because someone else gets away with something does not mean you will get away with it. The same holds true for safe and unsafe behavior. It doesn't matter how many other employees have successfully committed an unsafe act or shortcut if you are the one injured. To prevent the accident, all it would take is to perform the behavior safely.

We learn by other's examples and that corporate actions speak louder than corporate policies. The actions of the corporate officers obviously show the true policy of companies having safety regulations which are not enforced. When you understand this concept of communication you begin to understand the meaning of the old cliché, "Actions speak louder than words." You also can see that it is important to, "Walk your talk."

Being An Inspiration To Others

One thing we have the privilege of doing during our lifetime is to inspire others. I know some of you feel your life isn't that inspiring which brings us to a concept I learned from Anthony Robbins. "You get to choose whether your life will serve as an example or a warning." It is your decision how you will behave. If you do things safely you serve as an example to others of how to do it right, an excellent model for others to copy so they can also achieve excellence.

While a member of the Staff of Anthony Robbins' Life Mastery seminar in Hawaii I had the opportunity along with fifty members of my team to participate in an exercise designed to allow you to stretch the limits of your comfort zone. The particular exercise was to climb a fifty-foot telephone pole, stand on top of it and then jump seven feet across to a trapeze. Of course, you are attached to a safety harness but it is still exciting and for some people frightening. I am not afraid of heights and have done other "breaking through barrier" activities such as fire walking several times. (Just try and explain to safety professionals how to safely walk across a fifteen foot bed of hot coals barefoot.) I knew I would be able to climb the pole and reach the top. I didn't know if I would be able to jump far enough to grip the trapeze, but that did not matter to me. I had as my objective that I would climb successfully and make the jump attempt to the best of my ability. I'm sure you have had similar situations when you faced a task that was no big deal to you. You knew you could accomplish it and you just went ahead and did it.

My turn to climb arrived and I donned the safety harness and helmet and began my ascent. After going twenty feet I was winded due to my weight. I stopped and told my partner on the ground that I was fine. I didn't want it to be mistakenly concluded that I was stuck due to fear but understood that I was only catching my breath. After a few moments of pole hugging I decided if I waited any longer some people might be concerned so I continued on. I must have looked like a giant Koala bear as I hugged the pole. I got to about forty feet and had to rest again as I was winded. Having done my imitation of a Koala bear for the second time I continued to the top. A fellow safety professional suggested I looked like a giant tootsie pop in my red shirt and blue shorts atop this pole. When my waist was at the top of the pole I realized as I had on the ground that from this point onward I would have to let go of the pole in order to stand on top of it. This is quite a powerful metaphor. Just as I am sure you realize that after you have safety meetings and training sessions you ultimately have to let go and rely on the effectiveness of your communication to motivate your employees to work safely even when no one is watching.

Something magical happened after the climb. I noticed that many more people than usual came over to congratulate me on my successful climb to the top. I certainly appreciated the attention and thanked them for their comments. This continued for some time and then one of my team members came to me, held me by the shoulders and said, "Thank you. If I hadn't seen you climb to the top I wouldn't have been able to do it myself." Now I was getting really pumped up by all the praise but I began to discover that something significant had happened. I had been an inspiration to many other people watching. I hadn't done anything special in my opinion but apparently what I did had a major impact on a large group of people. I would guess that fifty to one hundred people congratulated me over the course of the next day. I thanked them but wondered inside what I had done that was unique or special. The next day someone shared with me that they had been standing next to the gentleman who owned the pole climbing company. He told me that the owner was truly moved as he watched me climb to the top. He shared with me that no one of my size had ever made it to the top. It was then that I realized by doing something ordinary in an excellent fashion I could have a positive impact on others. I am sure that you have had the same opportunity as safety professionals. The routine events of your day may be life changing to someone else.

At the other end of the spectrum you could choose to be a warning sign on the road of life to let others know the results of choosing to behave in an unsafe way. The choice is yours to make.

Be A Student Of Excellence - Look For Similarities

It is extremely valuable to study and read about successful people in general and specifically people who are in your own field of endeavor. By watching them either in books or in person you are exposed to a myriad of possibilities. You know that if they can do it so can you.

Keep in mind, also, it is vital to look for the similarities between them and you in order to achieve success. Too many people in the world today see successful people and say, "They are different from me, I could never do that." They are now dooming themselves and wiping out the value they have attained by watching successful people. If you look for ways you are similar, you will find solutions for your problems and see possibilities rather than exceptions. Look for people within your own company who work safely and people who are effective communicators and copy their strategies. Meet with safety professionals from other companies in your industry and find out what works for them and use it. The ways to improve yourself by modeling others' behavior are limitless.

Chapter 7

Giving and Receiving Feedback

"Everything works and nothing works.
It all depends on the context."
-- John W. Drebinger Jr.

Questions To Enhance Your Reading

1. What ideas in this chapter can I use to improve the safe behavior of myself and those with whom I work?

2. What positive behaviors do I know about each person I work around?

3. Who could I teach these techniques to in order to multiply my effectiveness?

4. Who should correct unsafe behaviors?

Safety Coaches

If we care about the safety of ourselves and others we must be willing to give and receive information about safe and unsafe behaviors. Strangely, it seems that it is difficult to tell someone something good as well as tell them about something they are doing wrong. This is evidenced by the fact that employees constantly report that managers very seldom give them praise. If we are uncomfortable giving praise, I wonder how much more difficult it is to offer a corrective comment.

Since I believe in taking personal responsibility, I need to make it easier for others to correct me when they observe me doing something unsafe or see me in a hazardous situation. The problem is that in our society it isn't natural or acceptable to correct others' behavior so I know they aren't likely to do so. Therefore, I would not benefit from their awareness of my situation. I began to look for a model where we expect people to give us critical input. I thought of coaching. We expect a coach to give us input. As you know, I am committed to constant improvement. Because of this, I hired a speech coach to show me how I could improve my presentations. We met and she watched me speak. She listened and watched videos of my presentations. After all of this, which I was paying her for, imagine if she were to say to me, "John, I think everything you are doing is great! I can't think of any way to make it better." How happy do you think I would have been to write her a check for her coaching? Obviously, I expected her to make suggestions and help me make the improvements she suggested.

Sports coaches are people we always want feedback from. If you have a child in a sports program you know how much difference a great coach can make in their performance. In fact, if the coach ignores your child you are disappointed because you know they won't improve as quickly or dramatically.

What I suggest is that you consider asking those around you to be your safety coach. Use whatever term with which you are comfortable. Perhaps, you might tell someone that you would appreciate it if they watch out for you and if they ever notice you near a hazard or doing something unsafe you would appreciate their input. Now, when they notice something they will be more comfortable telling you because they know you expect their comments.

Giving Feedback to Others

Many people have studied how to give feedback so that the person receiving it will be most likely to act on the comments. Ironically, the other half of the communication formula has been ignored. What can we do to make it comfortable to give feedback? The reason this is important is that people avoid that which is uncomfortable. I believe that people actually care about their fellow employees, their friends, and associates. I know that they would never want to see them injured because they failed to warn them of a hazard. The desire to help is overshadowed by the fear that they will not be appreciated for their input. Given this problem, I looked for a solution. What I came up with are ways you can inform someone of their behavior or risky situation and still feel good about it.

The first one came to me as I was doing my presentation, Ensure Your Safety. An audience member

was on stage with me and I noticed their shoelace was
untied. Now I had a dilemma. Do I point this out in front
of the entire audience or do I wait for later? The problem
was that the person was going to have to walk up some
stairs to get to their seat and tripping on a shoelace in this
situation could cause an injury. What I did and what you
can do is to ask the person, "Would you like me to watch
out for your safety?" In this case, the person said, "What?"
and I repeated, "Would you like me to watch out for your
safety?" They paused and said yes. I told him that their
shoe was untied and the person sat in the front row and
tied it before returning to their seat. I felt comfortable
because I had asked them if they wanted the input and
knew they wanted it.

Another technique is great if you are dealing with
someone who has more experience, seniority, or is higher
on the organizational chart than you. This technique uses
the phrase, "As you know..." For example, if you saw
someone lifting something that they should have help with
you could approach them and say, "As you know, you need
some help lifting that." This statement gives the person
credit for knowing what is supposed to be done but it
reminds them at that moment it is necessary in order to be
safe. They can respond and say, "I knew that. I was just
coming to get you."

We should encourage our fellow employees to seek
out input. If we don't ask for input we will never improve.
A great example of this occurred when I was speaking at
NASA's Johnson Space Center in Houston, Texas. I had
received enthusiastic feedback from the people who hired
me as well as my audiences. I decided to ask for some
input from one of the top people at the center. I asked
them if there was anything that would improve the
presentation for them. Their response was that it would be
helpful to summarize the key points right at the end of my
presentation. I went back to my hotel room and thought
how I could do that most effectively. I wrote the key points
to this feedback technique on a piece of paper and realized

that was the answer. I fired up my laptop computer and did the layout so it would fit on a business card. A quick trip to an office supply store and a few minutes at Kinkos and I had my prototype for the next day's presentation. The Safety Cards were a hit and I developed them into a new product I could offer my clients to enhance my message. If you would like to see a sample of these cards you can find them on my website www.drebinger.com They are in a section titled Training Resources and Products.

Receiving Feedback From Others

We also need to teach people how to receive feedback. After all, I can ask everyone to be my safety coach but if I sneer at them the first time they warn me about a hazard or behavior I will teach them to never do it again. People are very smart and they learn quickly. There is much truth to the saying, "Actions speak louder than words." When someone tells me about an unsafe behavior I need to thank them and let them know I appreciate that they cared enough about me to let me know. In addition, many companies have seen the wisdom of using behavior-based safety. One element of many behavior-based programs is some form of observation of one worker by another. This is done with the consent and awareness of the person being observed. I have heard from many employees that they feel uncomfortable doing the observation. It intrigues me that the hesitation is on the part of the observer and not the person being observed. Because of this, I encourage the person being observed to inform the observer that they are genuinely interested in their feedback and appreciate their taking time to do the observation. It is also helpful to have the person being observed ask some questions after the observation. They should inquire if anything was noticed that they could improve on. Even the best strive to be better. In either case, be sure to thank the person doing the observation. By the way, I learned years ago that a great way to thank someone is to thank their supervisor. You might want to take a moment to let their supervisor know you thought they did a thorough job doing their observation. If you really want to improve safety, let their supervisor know they helped you avoid an injury when they gave you feedback that you were doing something hazardous or were in danger.

The Magic Of Sandwich Style Criticism

There comes a time in everyone's life when they must offer criticism or correction of behavior which is unacceptable. There is a technique you can use to increase the effectiveness of the criticism or correction you offer to others. In order to facilitate change it is important to offer the criticism as soon as possible after the incorrect behavior is observed. The unconscious mind of an individual is most open to effective criticism within five minutes of the event being discussed. This makes it crucial that supervisors, employees, or managers learn to act quickly to teach people the safe way to perform their work.

Why Multiply Your Effectiveness

How much would your effectiveness as a safety professional be improved if most of the employees and supervisors in the workforce made it a point to correct unsafe behavior whenever they saw it occurring? How many accidents would be avoided if such correction resulted in safe behaviors?

No company could remain competitive if it had to hire enough safety professionals to be available to watch all employees personally during the entire workday. Likewise, as a safety professional it is impossible for you to be the eyes and ears watching out for everyone. Even if you could it might not be the most effective way to change behaviors.

Daily, your employees and supervisors notice others performing unsafe acts (the greatest cause of all accidents). What a tragedy it is that fellow workers see the foundation for an accident and because they are not willing to risk rejection they say nothing to the employee. How many times has an accident occurred and you hear someone say, "I saw that person do that behavior just the other day." Or the comment is made, "I'm not surprised, since he or she does that all the time. It's no wonder they finally got hurt."

People in our society are hesitant to offer correction or suggestions for change for fear people will not appreciate it or be upset with them. In order to overcome this you can remind employees that they need to remember how much they really care about their fellow workers. For many people, their friends are those they work with and even if they have no social connection with others at their place of work they probably do care about them. In my seminars, I ask the question, "What is the opposite of love?" The most common response is "hate". I then point out that apathy is the true opposite of love. Employees really discover how much they care about each other when a disabling or fatal injury occurs. I have found that people go out of their way to help the families affected by the accident. If we really care about others, we need to take action to avoid the injury in the first place. I then remind employees that to ignore a fellow worker's unsafe behavior is the most unloving response we can make. In order for people to actually take action you must give them tools which make it easier for them to successfully help their fellow employees. Your employees are more likely to correct others' behavior when they have been taught a method they feel comfortable using. You can multiply your effectiveness by giving employees and supervisors tools which will make it easy, comfortable and effective to change the way people work.

"Science may have found a cure for most evils, but it has found no remedy for the worst of them all - the apathy of human beings."

-- Helen Keller

Sandwich Style Criticism

    One tool used to correct inappropriate behavior and teach correct safe behavior is a concept called "Sandwich Style Criticism". This is an effective and inoffensive technique to correct unsafe behavior that will make a difference. In order to maximize the effectiveness of criticism it is best to use a particular formula to present the suggestion or correction. Sandwich Style Criticism uses a three part conversation to correct behaviors.

    •Positive comment
    •Correction
    •Positive comment

    First, point out something positive to the person, either your appreciation for how well they do their job, something you like about them or the way they deal with others. Second, mention the behavior, which must be modified and third, point out another positive item. This sandwiching of the correction between the two positives allows the person to feel good about themselves, which increases the likelihood they will accept the correction and make the right changes. When you begin with something positive the employee is feeling great because you have shown that your intention is to reinforce or support them. We all like to hear compliments about ourselves. In fact, one of the most common complaints employees in this country have is that they never get complimented by management, they only receive criticism. This technique is all the more powerful because of this phenomenon. When the positive comment begins the employee opens all of their listening senses. They want to hear more and you really have their attention. This prevents them from going on the defensive and instantly turning you off and as a result never hearing what you have to say. Now that they are fully committed to listening you make the comment about the behavior to be corrected. Be thorough but as brief as possible. If you go too long it dilutes the effect of the opening positive comment. Finally, you end on a positive note, which once again opens up their listening channels and keeps them from going on the defensive. This allows them to feel good which also increases their desire to improve and receive more of this much wanted praise.

An effective alteration of the above formula whenever possible is to make the middle section a description of the desired behavior rather than focusing on the incorrect behavior. Denis Waitley points out that people move towards the predominate thought and therefore telling them what you want them to do is much more effective. In the field of safety we are sometimes forced to state the prohibited behavior or the hazard, but please add to it the behavior you want in its place.

An example might be, "Hey, Bob, I really appreciate how quickly you get the shipments out. It really makes a difference to our clients. I just noticed you lifting that box without bending your knees and I'm afraid if you continue to lift that way you will injure your back. As important as you are to our operation, I would hate to see you miss work because of an injury. Besides, the other employees look to you for leadership. They like you and you set the pace out here."

To change this to a positive direction in the middle you could say, "Do you have a minute to talk about lifting techniques? I wanted to review them with you," instead of pointing out you observed him lifting improperly. In most cases, they will figure out something they did precipitated the discussion but they do not have to offer an excuse and they are less likely to be offended.

One other fine tuning point, most people will catch on quickly that every time you pay them a compliment it is followed with a correction. In order to overcome this, make it a point to compliment them occasionally without correction. Then they will not build up a resistance to the technique.

How To Come Up With A Positive List

In order to be ready to correct someone doing something inappropriate or unsafe you must be prepared with a list of positive things you can comment on. In order to do this you should make a list of those people who work around you and those whom you would like to add to your circle of responsibility. You need to plan ahead and as you walk around your facility make notes about what employees are doing right. This set of notes becomes your resource for sandwich criticism. Once you have a list you can record it in a small pocket size notebook available at most stationery stores. You should carry it with you during the day and ask yourself the question "What is positive or valuable that I could write down about **(Person's Name Inserted Here)**?" When an idea comes to your mind write it down next to or under their name. Continue this process until you have at least three and hopefully, five positive statements about each person. Now you are armed and ready to practice "Sandwich Style Criticism" effectively. Some people might think this is too much work to keep track of but by writing it down you don't have to remember all the details. Whenever you find yourself asking the question, "Doesn't this seem like too much trouble?" stop and ask the question, "If this is all I had to do to protect someone from getting hurt would I do it?" If you find yourself stuck and unable to find anything positive to say ask yourself, "I know I can't think of anything positive about this person but if I could what would it be?"

You tend to see what you focus on and so it is useful to prepare for sandwich style criticism by observing and writing down positive behaviors of employees for recognition when needed.

In addition to having a list for sandwich style criticism, your opinion of the people around you is likely to change. This change in attitude will affect the way you communicate with them in a very positive way.

Also, how many times have you heard from employees and know from your own experience that praise by management is oftentimes nonexistent? Even if you are an outstanding manager and already point out to employees what a great job they are doing, imagine the effects of pointing out their safe behavior. They will realize that you put safety in the important role it deserves. It makes them feel that safe work habits are another way of receiving praise, instead of always being a burden. Additionally, it reinforces the procedures and policies your company has regarding safety.

Planning Ahead For Spontaneity
In the safety field we always want to have employees ask the question, "What if?" in order to anticipate hazards and reasons for which they need personal protective equipment. We, as safety professionals, need to ask ourselves, "What if we see an unsafe behavior? What are we willing to do? Are we prepared to correct it in the most effective fashion?

People often marvel when an entertainer uses an ad-lib that sounds brilliant and which appears to be a spontaneous response to some unexpected comment from a member of the audience. Nothing could be further from the truth. The best comedians plan their ad-libs and keep track of what gags work and in what situations. When the opportunity arises they have already "written" a response to what might happen during their routine. We need to be as clever. Planning ahead for those opportunities to change behavior is critical to our success. Having standard lines, which we have practiced will make the comments seem spontaneous even when they are not. Making notes about what employees are doing right prepares your resource when needed for sandwich style criticism.

Chapter 8

Creative Ideas

"Ideas, the children of your mind may appear childish or insignificant at first but written down, nurtured and given respect can grow into the revelations of your tomorrow's."
-- John W. Drebinger Jr.

Questions To Enhance Your Reading

1. What ideas in this chapter can I use to improve the safe behavior of myself and those with whom I work?

2. How can I get myself out of a stuck state?

3. How can I get others out of a stuck state?

4. What actions could I take to increase my imagination?

How People Get Into A Stuck State

Have you ever experienced a time in your life when you were having trouble coming up with an idea? Have you ever observed someone at work saying, "I can't do that" and then nothing happened, or you said, "I can't do that" and find that you're stuck? What did you just do to yourself? You just put yourself into a type of trance. A trance can be defined in this case as a focused state. Whenever you are concentrating on something to the exclusion of everything else you are in a trance. Trance states are very simple and in fact people put themselves into a trance several times each day. You put yourself and others into a trance or a focused state by saying, "I don't know how to do that." In this example the focus is on what you can not do. Usually when you say that, your unconscious mind which is very suggestible and willing to comply says, "OK, I understand you don't know how to do that." Your unconscious mind wants to remain consistent with the conscious mind so it will sabotage any solution you may try so that the first command you gave it, (i.e. I can't do that) will remain true.

Getting Someone Out Of A Stuck State

As a member of the faculty of the Los Angeles Chapter of the National Safety Council's Training Institute, I saw an example of this. A person was there who wanted to learn how to generate creative ideas for safety meetings. I knew this because at the beginning of the day I asked people why they had come to the training session that day. I asked what desired outcome they wanted from the course and the answer was, "I am just not creative, I can't come up with any new ideas." This, by the way, was stated as the person's identity, "I am just not creative." I could have said, "Oh, sure you can, you are great at safety ideas, you can come up with ideas." Since I was just told by the person that they couldn't come up with any ideas, if I didn't acknowledge that belief, I would get a negative response. Someone in this situation might respond to themselves internally, "You're not listening!" Then they would search for ways to convince me of their belief. In addition to being guilty of not listening I have challenged this person's identity. That is sure to create a greater degree of resistance. The negative side of this is that the belief is being reinforced as the attempt to convince me is taking place. The brain is now committed to convincing me that they really don't know what to do. That reinforces the state which is negative.

I Know You Don't Know But If You Did Know?

To move a person out of that state is a simple thing to do. You can get somebody to come up with an idea even when they are blocked. That someone could even be you! When someone says, "I don't know how!" you reply, "I know you don't know how, but, if you did know, how would you do it?" That does two things for the person. First off, you don't put them into a trance or an "I don't know" cycle. You have acknowledged their belief which makes them realize they have been heard. The other thing it does is create an idea or concept of possibility. It presupposes that it is possible to do it in such a way that the conscious mind will have no objection. One illustration of this concept occurred in the 1950's. At the time no runner had been able to break the four minute mile. It was an invisible wall that no one had been able to break through. Suddenly a man named Roger Bannister came along and broke the four minute mile, proving it was possible. The most interesting part of this story is that in that very same year 38 other runners broke the four minute mile. Now what had happened? Did they all of a sudden become better runners? No! Their brains now knew that it was in fact possible to achieve this new record and then they could do it. Their brains said, "We can do this," and they did.

I read once that the director of the National Transportation Safety Board said, "We should have zero accidents this year." Jay Leno, that evening made a joke about it saying that we should have one big wreck each year. What was interesting is that the director had a very valid point. The key is that in order to achieve something you must first believe that it is possible to do. The whole point is if the whole industry can grasp the idea then it is possible to go years upon years without a plane crashing. Remember that as soon as Roger Bannister broke the four-minute mile people thought it was possible. The director at the National Transportation Safety Board made a statement which shows he believes it is possible to have zero accidents. He had caught the vision and from there he could take measures to make it happen. Unfortunately, several people in the room said, "No, it's not." There are some people who believe it is impossible to have a one hundred percent safe airline, given the current economy, the competition and the deregulation. However, if the director had said, "That's right, it's not possible, but if it were possible how would you do it?" he would have opened the door to their being able to envision what he knew was possible.

You see at that point you stop arguing with the person's model of the world, the representation they have in their brain. As a result, they realize they have been heard and respected and they are now willing to deal with the imagined possibility of what it would take to accomplish the task. You open up the possibility. A Roger Bannister shows up on the scene and you know what happens. Now your brain says, "OK, I know it's not possible but if it was what would I do?" Then it goes into the problem solving mode. Whenever you find yourself saying, "I can't," or "I don't know how," agree with yourself. Say, "That's right, I don't know but if I did what would I do?" It even works when you know you are doing it to yourself.

Back to my training class in Los Angeles when I asked one person, "What do you want to learn today?" That person said, "I don't know how to come up with any creative ideas for safety meetings." I replied, "I know you don't know but if you did know what would be a good safety idea you could use at your next meeting?" A chuckle resulted and everyone else laughed because I had just taught this technique. The reply was, "I don't know." I said, "I know you don't know but if you did know how would you do it?" Again, the answer was, "I really don't know." I replied, "I know you really don't know but if you did know what would you do?" Then I just shut up and there was quiet as thinking took over. Keep in mind that I had already taught the class this technique. It was just as if a magician told you how a trick worked and then performed it and it still amazed you. Inside of five minutes half of a page filled with new ideas for making safety meetings more interesting. I should point out that these ideas were generated with no one in the class making any helpful suggestions since this was an exercise in coming up with ideas in your own mind. As a result, the person had ideas that they knew would work with their employees. These were ideas that would fit the work place and the needs of that company. Just moments before, the person thought they were not creative and were not capable of doing what they had just accomplished. How did the person get to that point? Not by my saying, "Sure you can do it." The difficulty with this phrase is it locks a person's brain into this state of being stuck. The secret is to agree with someone that they can't do it and then give them the key to opening up the possibility that they can do it. You tell them you know they can't do it but if they could how would they and then wait for the results. When they do accomplish it, you can even teach them the technique so that they can continue to use it on themselves. It is a tremendous tool you can use in any area. You ask yourself the questions, "How can we improve our safety record next year? How can we achieve better results?" You say, "I don't know how we can get better, but if we could, how would we do it?" You can do this by talking to yourself. First, agree with yourself and you will discover a big difference in your results. Each one of us is capable of putting on interesting and effective training meetings if we take the time to ask the right question: "How can I improve the effectiveness of my training?"

Activities You Can Do To Improve Imagination

Whenever you want to excel at something find an expert and find out how they do it. Once you discover their strategy and are able to copy it, you can achieve the same level of success or better. When it comes to imagination, children have to be the world's greatest experts. In an instant they can pretend two chairs covered with a blanket is a massive secret cave or even a spaceship. If you want to imagine things, do some of the things children do. Ask questions, look at something upside down or inside out, take an object and make up a new and different use for it. Take some blank paper and draw something, (I know you can't draw well but if you could what would you draw?) Thinking like a child is a way to help your imagination grow. Children grow quickly because they are insatiably curious. In fact, growing is one of the things you must be committed to if you want to improve your ability to imagine. Children are fearless and at times they take risks. They risk looking silly or making a mistake. Try playing make-believe or try writing with the opposite hand than you normally use. Try drawing with one hand and then the other.

"Study as if you were going to live forever; live as if you were going to die tomorrow."

-- **Maria Mitchell**

Read! Read! Then read some more. The average American stops reading after high school except non-fiction or informational reading. Read something just to expand your horizons. Try talking to yourself consciously, talk to the trees, animals or whatever you like. If they answer then you really have supercharged your imagination. You know you are in big trouble when you talk to yourself, argue with yourself and lose the argument. Walt Disney looked to nature for inspiration. Take a moment to play and see your world through the eyes of a child. In fact, it's never too late to have a happy childhood if you learn to act like a child and who knows what life saving ideas you might originate.

An Example Of The Evolution Of A Training Technique

I began to develop the balloon trick to illustrate the concept of possibility thinking. My original outcome for the effect was to show that oftentimes people won't even try something they haven't seen done before. I soon discovered I could use the effect to show how people unconsciously model others in order to do what they do. Consistently, after doing the trick I noticed that when I handed the balloon and needle to the person they would always take the balloon and put the needle in just at the same spot I did. I did not instruct them on how to do the trick I merely did it. They unconsciously modeled my strategy and as a result most people would successfully accomplish the trick on their first attempt. I then caught the vision of a new employee or someone with less experience watching an experienced worker and unconsciously learning how they do that job. If the procedure the experienced worker was using was unsafe or incorrect the new employee was most likely going to model the other employee's behavior even if it contradicted company policy. We learn what the real rules are by watching what others do. When the local custom is different than what we were taught we will adapt to that in order to become more accepted.

**"If you have knowledge,
    let others light their candles in it."**

-- Margaret Fuller

Sharing Ideas With Others

One great thing about the safety business is that safety professionals are willing to share because everyone benefits. Several of my clients make it a point to send their safety chairman to visit other safety meetings held within their company to check what other divisions are doing. It is also possible to contact some of your competitors and ask to visit their meetings and in return invite them to yours. In many cases this would help keep workers compensation costs down if in a given industry we all worked together.

If you are interested in sharing your ideas with others or you have an effective story which illustrates a safety lesson I am providing a vehicle for doing this in a new book I am currently compiling. If you would like to share your ideas with others please read the information on page 155 then contact us. We will help share your effective ideas and stories with others and give you credit for your creativity and effort.

Chapter 9

What's In A Word?

"What's in a name? That which we call a rose by any other name would smell as sweet."
-- Romeo and Juliet, William Shakespeare

Questions To Enhance Your Reading

1. What ideas in this chapter can I use to improve the safe behavior of myself and those with whom I work?

2. What powerful negative words could I change to neutral or negative without the intensity?

3. What positive meanings could I put on things to change how I feel about them?

4. How easy can I make something by changing the words I describe it with?

Language and Thinking

I heard at a seminar I attended that the language you speak affects the way you think. People from different countries using different languages will think about the same physical item differently. I was fascinated by this so I began to ask those people I met in my speaking engagements around this country about their thoughts and their language. I asked people who were proficiently bilingual enough to think in both languages. Consistently, they told me the thinking process they use is different depending in what language they are thinking at that moment. Perhaps that explains one of the reasons we don't always have an easy time understanding the behavior of people in other countries around the world. We both witness the same event but think about it with a different set of words. So what does this have to do with you as a safety professional? Well, the words you use have a strong effect on your thinking or response to the world around you. You can use those words to help you change the responses to what you want.

Words - The Keys To Your Thoughts

In addition to affecting the way you think, the words you use can limit your ability to think and be creative. I grew up in Southern California and the only snow I ever experienced was in the mountains surrounding Los Angeles. I had only one word for snow. When I went camping in the snow one weekend I developed several more distinctions about snow and added those adjectives to the word snow to increase my ability to think, conceptualize and communicate about snow. I knew there was wet snow which was great for making snow balls and dry snow which was useless for such games but less messy if you had to sit down in it for any length of time. Even with this expanded vocabulary for snow I did not have the same resources for thinking about snow that someone living in the Arctic would have. Their life depends upon accurately describing and making distinctions about the environment in which they live. When I lived in Minnesota for three years my vocabulary for snow increased as did my conceptual limits for it. My wife and I had taken up cross country skiing and we would spend many evenings and weekends out in the snow. We defined snow in relationship to the effect it had on our skiing. Our particular skis required a special wax to allow you to gain forward motion. As a result we labeled the snow in relation to the type of wax needed for the best traction and glide while skiing. Green snow was dry and you would use a hard green wax in order to not clump up snow on the bottom of the skis. If there was a fresh snow and it was twenty degrees below zero we called it light green snow, not because it had changed color but rather the wax we needed was light green in color and harder. In the springtime we would ski in yellow snow. No, it wasn't what you are thinking. Yellow snow is wet melting spring snow and in order to get traction you use a very sticky yellow wax henceforth the name yellow snow. By just reading this story your vocabulary about snow has increased and you, too, can think differently about snow.

That is the beauty of reading books regularly, you increase your vocabulary and therefore your ability to think.

Change The Meaning - Change The Feeling

Words are used by us as a medium in which to think. When you analyze something it is usually done with words. In addition to limiting what and how you think about something, words affect the way you feel or the level of intensity with which you experience life. For example, I fly over one hundred thousand miles every year and I meet many people who "hate" flying. They are not afraid to fly they just dislike the experience. I do not enjoy all aspects of flying but I know it is an unavoidable part of my career so I use language to enhance my enjoyment of it. Instead of feeling "cooped up and trapped" for several hours I describe it as "being waited on and taken care of" for several hours. My emotional state is going to be much more resourceful when I have to communicate with others because I am enjoying the experience instead of being miserable. Too often when I hear safety professionals discuss difficulties to be overcome they attach the phrases, "It is really tough" or "It's impossible" to their remarks. When they use such negatively charged words you can see how the solution seems so far away and out of their grasp.

Words You Say To Yourself

If they controlled the use of their internal conversation they might say instead, "It's a challenge" or "It is really interesting." These words have less intensity and therefore the problem is much more likely to be solved. When you understand that your choice of vocabulary affects what you can think about, you can use this to your advantage. What would happen if you artificially altered the vocabulary you use to change the way you think about something? If you really want to find yourself using words to change the way you think, speak in terms of the desired effect. Your unconscious mind begins to move in the direction that you speak to yourself and others. If you are constantly focused on the negative and the things you have not figured out yet you will develop a state of being depressed. If instead, you talk as if it were "easy" to accomplish the things you need to do your unconscious mind will fulfill that result as easily.

"There are two ways of meeting difficulties. You alter the difficulties or you alter yourself to meet them."

-- Phyllis Bottome

Choose the words you use intentionally when you talk to yourself because they, in addition to the questions you ask, will direct your life and your communication with others. You might consider combining the appropriate physiology and tonality to the way you reframe something in order to increase its effect. Remember, you have the power to change the meaning something has for you by changing the words you use to label it. The content with which you are dealing does not have to change, only the meaning you give it. By changing its meaning your approach to it will be altered considerably. For example, if you refer to something as a horrendous problem it is certainly going to be more difficult than if you look at it as an intriguing puzzle. As safety professionals we must realize that the words we choose can increase the effectiveness of what we communicate.

"The real voyage of discovery consists not in seeing new landscapes but in having new eyes."

-- Marcel Proust

Chapter 10

Outcomes

"Discover your uniqueness and exploit it in service to others and you are guaranteed success, prosperity and happiness."

-- Larry Winget

Questions To Enhance Your Reading

1. What ideas in this chapter can I use to improve the safe behavior of myself and those with whom I work?

2. What specific outcomes do I have for the safety of the people around me?

3. What would make an outcome compelling to me?

4. What is the concept of "act as if"? When should I use it?

Outcomes, Yours and Theirs

Outcomes are crucial to effective communication. Try looking at outcomes from two perspectives. First, your own outcomes and second, the outcomes of your audience or individuals with whom you are communicating. You must know your expected outcomes in order to master the words, tonality and physiology you will use to get your point across. Knowing the outcome of your audience will increase your ability to meet their needs and therefore succeed. When these outcomes are compatible, you will be able to achieve significant results. If they are not, your ability to be flexible and do whatever it takes will be very necessary in order to be successful in your communication.

Leaders Have Specific Outcomes

I had the privilege of hearing Norman Schwarzkopf speak about leadership and achieving objectives. He pointed out that the most critical thing related to success is that you need to know before you start what criteria will determine the measure of your success. You must identify your outcome prior to taking action. In the Desert Storm action it had been decided ahead of time that getting Sadam Hussein out of Kuwait was the objective. In fact, the operation would be a success even without continuing on into Baghdad. The political nature of the alliance which made up the multinational force would not have allowed such a goal. Therefore, the political objective for the military action was clear and it allowed them to accurately measure their success against a standard. They knew when they had achieved success.

How many times have you given an employee a task and failed to let them know how they would measure their success in completing the task? However, if you convey in advance that they will be successful when they accomplish these specific things, it will then be easy for them and for you to measure their results.

Programming Your Brain To Achieve Your Outcomes

Ten years ago I was going to Florida for the first time and because I have been a fan of the United States space program and NASA for years I arranged two extra days so I could take any tours of the Kennedy Space Center that were available. I was excited as I rode the bus around the space center seeing all the places you have seen on television when they cover a launch. On one of the tours you stop just outside a fenced circle next to either pad 39a or 39b. We exited the bus and were allowed to take pictures. I stood there in awe realizing I was looking at the spot where we as humans stepped off of the earth and stepped onto the moon. The pads that had launched the Apollo spacecraft had been modified to launch the space shuttle. Looking up at the massive launch tower I was thrilled but I also realized that I had to see more. I decided right then and there that someday I was going to stand on the launch tower.

Perhaps you have something you are passionate about such as improving the safe behaviors of people with whom you work. Once you decide that you want to improve safety results you are on the way. Making a decision puts our brain into action but you are much more likely to hit a target or outcome that has real clarity. I, without knowing it, programmed my brain for success that afternoon. The technique is simple but profound and is easy for you to use in achieving the results you want. I knew exactly what it would look like, sound like, feel like, smell like, and taste like when I would be standing on that tower. I knew I would see the Atlantic ocean to my left. In front of me would be the old launch sites and looking down I would see the flame trench. To the right I would see the Vehicle Assembly Building four miles away. I also knew I would be attentively listening to someone telling me all about what I was standing on and looking at. I knew I would feel the wind blowing across the cape and through my clothes. I also knew that I would smell the ocean in the air and probably even taste it. What I had done without realizing it was program my computer using the five input devices we as humans have. Everything you have stored in your mind has been taken in through your five senses. Just as a computer uses a keyboard and a mouse as input devices our brain has these five input devices. By making the outcome sensory specific you can chart the course that will take you where you want to go.

Since that day ten years ago I developed my speaking career and finally had the opportunity to do a training session at the Kennedy Space Center for the safety team. When my presentation was over they had promised to take me on a tour. We went to the orbital processing facility where they get the space shuttle (orbiter) ready for the next mission. I was so excited I was almost in outer space myself.

Reach Higher Levels of Performance By Stretching Your Own Outcomes

My outcome for this trip was to be able to stand on the launch tower and also to get close enough to one of the space shuttles to be able to touch it. After checking in we walked under the Space Shuttle Atlantis and I looked up at the tiles that protect it from the heat of re-entry, you could see the ones that had just been replaced and the ones with marks from previous missions. It was incredible and a dream come true. We walked upstairs and I stood at the nose of the orbiter where I met Mike who was in charge of this facility. He told me it was too bad I had not been there the previous week. I asked why figuring that something special had happened. He said that had I been there one week earlier they could have taken me aboard the shuttle onto the actual flight deck. I was stunned, I was still thrilled to have the privilege of being there but I realized that I had set my outcomes too low. Have you ever set your sights too low because you didn't know or believe something was possible. It is easy in the safety profession to get discouraged unless you focus on your ultimate outcome and allow you brain to find a way to achieve it. I decided at that moment that I would always dream the biggest dreams and set the highest outcomes in order to experience life to its fullest. They did however tell me that when I came back to do some more training that they would get me on board.

We then drove out to launch pad 39a and drove up the ramp to the base of the launch tower. We entered the elevator and went to the two hundred fifty five foot level. I walked out of the elevator and what a beautiful view. I looked to my left and saw the Atlantic ocean. In front of me were the old launch sites and looking down I could see the flame trench. To the right I saw the Vehicle Assembly Building four miles away. Our escort at the pad was relating to us about the Apollo program and also explaining the structure we were on. I felt the wind blowing across the cape and through my clothes. I could smell the ocean in the air and even tasted it. I then looked down and watched a tour bus pull up and as the people got out to take photos and I realized that I had been there ten years earlier. Goose bumps went from my head to my toes as I realized I had achieved exactly what I programmed my brain to accomplish. You can achieve your outcomes by making them sensory specific.

Helping Others Reach Higher Standards By Stretching Your Own Outcomes

Remember, that they had promised on my next visit I would be able to go inside a space shuttle? Well, I returned several months later and this time as we went into the Orbital Processing Facility we were issued clean suits. After signing in we went through an air shower and then put on the special garments. I was then invited to climb on a small platform that went through the hatch and into the Space Shuttle Atlantis. It had just returned from a rendezvous with the space station Mir. I climbed a ladder and entered the flight deck where they allowed me to look through the windows to the cargo bay and explained the equipment on board. Our escort then asked if I would like to sit in the pilot's seat and proceeded to give me directions on how to accomplish this task. (The photo on the front cover is of me in the pilot's seat.) I sat there with the joy stick in one hand and I was thrilled. It was then that I discovered something else special. As I looked to my left my friend Jack was sitting in the commander's seat with a big smile on his face and it was then I realized in his career with NASA he had never taken the opportunity to go on board one of the space shuttles. I discovered that when we achieve our outstanding outcomes we get to bring along others we care about. This is especially true for us in the safety profession. When you are successful helping others to work safely they benefit as you achieve the safety outcomes you have programmed into your brain. As you raise your standards many people benefit.

Guidelines For An Achievable Outcome

State Your Outcome In the Positive

Not long ago I had the opportunity to help a client who wanted to overcome their fear of flying. The client had been given airfare and two weeks accommodations in Hawaii yet was absolutely afraid to fly. When we sat down to deal with this situation I asked what they wanted to achieve. I was asking for the desired outcome. The immediate response was, "I don't want to be afraid during the flight." I said that was fine but that it is difficult to achieve a negative outcome such as that. I asked if it were possible to wave a magic wand what would the experience of flying to Hawaii be like? The client told me enjoying the flight and having a good time would be just right. That was great! Now I had an outcome which was positive and achievable. After only two hours of work we achieved the desired outcome and as a result the flight and the entire trip were a big success. The client told me later that even the flights between islands on the smaller planes were enjoyable.

You have probably been faced with challenges where the outcome you set for yourself was for something not to happen or some other negative representation of a goal. The difficulty you experienced may have been a result of not having a positive goal. Knowing this you can learn in this chapter to develop outcomes in such a way as to increase the likelihood of achieving them.

One summer I witnessed another example of why it is important to state your outcome in the positive. I observed lifeguards at a public pool and the effectiveness of their communication. A boy was running across the decking when the lifeguard yelled, "Don't run." The boy continued on at the same speed and jumped into the pool. Perhaps in his mind he wasn't running he was in the process of jumping. Later another lifeguard was on duty and when a boy was running they said, "Walk." Almost instantly the boy began to walk because it was easy to understand the desired behavior. Whenever possible state your outcomes and desired behaviors in the positive.

Be Specific In What You Want

In addition to being stated in the positive your outcomes must state specifically what you want.
For example:

- I want my employees to work safely.

- I want employees to follow all safety procedures.
- I want management committed to safety.
- I want employees committed to safety.
- I want a raise. (Not a safety goal but it is specific)

Take Into Account Their Current Behavior

With any journey you have a starting point and a destination. Knowing the destination is important but the instructions or specific steps you take in getting there are also determined by your starting point. Evaluate what the current behavior is then develop a plan to achieve the outcome. The more you know about where you are starting from will allow you to accurately develop a communication strategy that will yield results.

Outcomes Initiated and Maintained By You

The starting point includes your personal outcome. Can the outcome you have decided upon be initiated by you and maintained by you? If it can, you have much more control over its success. If it can't, then it merely means you must take that into account and involve others to achieve the results you must have.

Make Your Outcomes Sensory Specific

Remember what you learned in an earlier chapter about Representational Systems. When speaking about your outcomes it is important to remember that you use your senses to evaluate the world around yourself. Your brain represents the world using your senses through representational systems, so it is helpful to make your outcomes sensory based and measurable. What will I see when I achieve this outcome? What things will I hear from myself internally and from others externally when I achieve this outcome? What will it feel like when I have achieved this outcome? If there are smells or tastes associated with the outcome, they should be looked at in the same way. When you use these as ways to define your outcome your brain has a well-defined target and knows, just as a laser guided missile, when it has hit the well-defined target.

Is It Compelling?

Can you can think of something in your life that you decided you must have, whether it is a material possession, position or power. You know that you are willing to do whatever it takes to get what you want. The rule is that if you want something enough you will figure out how to achieve it. This is the same level you must achieve if you want to increase your effectiveness as a safety professional. What is the importance of it and what does it mean? You can make something more compelling by picturing in your mind the massive change which will be achieved.

Discover the power of possibility. Give your mind permission to open up and move forward because it knows it is possible. If you see it you can achieve it!! There are many examples throughout our history that illustrate how someone had a vision and led many others. John F. Kennedy saw us landing a man on the moon and it became a reality. Walt Disney saw Epcot and it became a reality. Sally Ride saw herself as an astronaut and became the first American woman in space. In each case, believing something was possible and seeing it as if it were completed, helped to make it a reality.

Likewise, there is danger in what you predict and what you see. If you imagine something won't work, it probably won't. Your unconscious mind will move towards the predominate image. You should always be sure you are imagining empowering possibilities.

You must make it compelling enough for your mind to create the result. See the outcome in the future. See yourself in the future with the outcome achieved.

"Whether you think you can or think you can't
**   - you are right."**

**   -- Henry Ford**

Determine Specific Evidence Of Achievement

There is specific evidence which lets you know when you have achieved your outcome. How do you know when you have achieved it? What specifically will you see, hear, and feel? Much of this you have already done by making the outcome sensory specific.

Is It What You Really Want?

You may have heard the admonition, "Be careful what you ask for you just might get it." That is exactly what this step is about. Are you willing to do whatever it takes to achieve your outcome and how will taking these actions affect the rest of your life? My friend, Bruce Wilkinson, tells his clients that they should set their policies and consequences for violating those policies as if their most valuable employee would violate the rule. If you have said you will take a particular course of action if someone violates a safety procedure, and then you do not administer the enforcement of it in a fair and equitable manner, you will destroy the outcome. This commitment is how you determine the difference between a wish and a desired compelling future. What do you have at stake in getting this outcome? What's in it for you? The more compelling you can make it the harder your brain will work to achieve it.

Who Is This Outcome Up To?

Is this outcome up to you? If it is, rise to the challenge and make it happen. If not, use your communication skills to enlist the help of others to do their part to make it happen. Is it initiated by you and maintained by you? Once again, if so, go and get it done. If not, what must you do to motivate others to do their part?

Do You Have A Choice Of Ways To Achieve It?

Is there more than one way to achieve your outcome? Flexibility is important in achieving outcomes. Remember the old saying, "There is more than one way to skin a cat." When in the past have you ever done this or something like this successfully? Do you know anyone who has achieved this outcome?

Is The First Step Specified And Achievable?

One of my performance mentors taught me that if you take action towards a goal within twenty four hours of setting that goal your chances for achieving it go up dramatically. You can probably think of situations where you took the first step and once you began, momentum instantly was achieved. Once you take action you seem to keep moving. For most people, the first step is the longest one of any journey they are taking.

Specify the first step necessary, take action and do it. Of course once you have started, it is useful to keep going so it is important that you have listed all the steps needed to achieve your outcome. Keep going down the list of steps until you accomplish what you want.

What Resources Do You Need To Achieve Your Outcome?

What resources do you have now and which ones will you need to achieve your outcome? When in the past have you ever done this or something like this successfully? Do you know anyone who has achieved this outcome?

Act As If

When have you heard this before? Once you have established an outcome using the above guidelines act as if you have achieved it. Your unconscious mind doesn't distinguish between imagination and reality. For example, Dr. Krasner has his students try the following exercise. Imagine a nice, big yellow lemon sitting on your desk. Imagine picking it up and taking a knife and cutting it in half. See the juice drip on the table. Now pick up one half of the lemon and bite into it. If you have done as I just asked I am sure you are puckering up just as if you had actually done it. The puckering your mouth is doing is based purely on imagination because you and I both know the only lemon on your table came from within your mind. When you acted as if you were biting into a lemon your salivary glands knew just what to do. The same is true for your outcomes. When you act as if you can achieve something your brain does the rest. It won't produce saliva for you but it will cause you to do the things which will direct you to achieve your outcome.

Some Fine Tuning Questions To Ask
- How will achieving this outcome affect your life?
- What is your purpose for achieving this outcome?
- What will you gain if you have it?
- What will you lose if you have it? (Sometimes gaining one thing means losing something else. If you have more to lose, your brain will make sure you will not achieve your outcome.)
- What will happen if you achieve this outcome?
- What will happen if you don't achieve it?
- What won't happen if you achieve it?
- What won't happen if you don't achieve your outcome?

Have you ever really looked at your outcomes in this manner before? Can you see reasons why some of your outcomes in the past haven't been achieved because these outcomes did not take any of the above into account? Practice developing outcomes for your safety meetings, your interaction with other people and whatever else you want to accomplish. You will find doing this will be enlightening and fun.

Chapter 11

Logistics

"Everything you do becomes what you make of it."

-- John W. Drebinger Jr.

Questions To Enhance Your Reading

1. What ideas in this chapter can I use to improve the safe behavior of myself and those with whom I work?

2. What are some situations where I could use a person's name to increase the effectiveness of my communication?

3. How can I make sure people observe my physiology when talking to groups?

4. What new ways could I present my material to increase its effectiveness?

The Magic Of One Word

Have you ever thought about the most important word in the world? As a safety professional you might think of safety or some related word, but that illustrates one of the challenges you face. In a diverse workplace you must be aware of your own biases which affect your ability to communicate. In my experience and according to many successful communicators a person's name is the most important word to them. When it really comes down to it, whether they like to admit it or not, people consider their own name to be the most important word to them. Have you ever noticed when you hear your name called out in a public place by someone you instantly turn around even when you know you are not the person to whom they are referring. You can be in a town where nobody knows you and when you hear your name called out you turn around, or at least your attention is diverted. That is the power your name has over you. Since we know it has this effect we should make use of it as effective communicators.

Knowing the power of a person's name allows me to use it to increase the effectiveness of my communication. One technique I have found useful when doing group presentations is to use a person's name whenever possible. It is helpful to have people make name plates at their seats big enough so that you can see it from your position in the room. When you are doing group presentations there are several advantages to this technique. First off, I can call people by name which is nice and I'm not embarrassed by not knowing somebody's name although I've already been introduced to them. Another thing I can do is quickly survey the room and notice if I have several people in the room with the same name thereby discovering which names are most common in the room. Armed with this information I use or call on those people. Every time I do I get the attention of everyone else in the room with the same name. In addition, if you notice someone's attention is not where you want it, you could call on them but that might point out to everyone in the room that you have lost them. Instead, whenever possible I will first call on someone in a different area with the same name. This grabs the attention of the other person and then I can call on them next thus keeping them involved and not embarrassing them or myself. You can increase the percentage of people in a room who are listening to you, if you use this little technique.

If you don't know anyone in the room and they don't have name tags there is another trick you can use. Select common names such as John, Mary, or some of the more common names in our culture or in the culture you are addressing. When you use those names you will have their attention. On the other hand, if you have people from other cultures and they have common names you are aware of, use one of them and suddenly their ears will perk up and they will be more attentive. If you know you've got people who are in different groups, cliques or work together in the same department you can use this to your advantage. I do many presentations for companies and I will observe the people in the room before I start or during breaks. People in a room will gather together in groups and I will utilize this phenomenon by picking someone from a group.

Suddenly the others in their group are watching very intently to see what I am going to do to their friend or co-worker. If you have groups of people in a room that you are dealing with picking one of them gives you a big advantage because you will have the attention of everyone else in that group.

Bad At Names? Here Is A Strategy That Works!

Years ago I worked as a District Scout Executive for the Boy Scouts of America. In the first district I served in Southern California I had a volunteer who was gifted at remembering people's names. He was known for always knowing everyone's name. As we dropped by businesses in town or as we walked by people on the street he called most people by using their correct name. I wanted to know how he did this so I asked him. He told me his secret. He said, "I guess." I was surprised and upon asking him if he was kidding he said, "Not really." His strategy was that when he saw someone he thought he knew he trusted the first name that his mind came up with. He learned to trust his unconscious mind which served him well. What happened when he was wrong? Nothing major, the person corrected him and they were not upset because they, like most people, don't believe they are good at names either so they did not expect him to be right. When he did get it right which was most of the time they were impressed. I used to say to people, "Excuse me, I forgot your name. What is it?" With that strategy I got one hundred percent of the names wrong and impressed no one.

When I tried his strategy it worked. I also changed my internal dialogue or self talk from saying, "I'm not good at names," to "I am good at names." My mind knew how to fulfill the self talk and now I am very good at names. I began by learning a strategy and "acting as if" I was good and it became true.

Recently someone I had not seen in over two years droped by to see my seminar. As he walked into the room I called him by name and he was impressed. Now what went on in my mind was interesting to me. His name came to my mind followed by doubt. I was afraid it was not correct but instead of listening to the doubt I trusted my unconscious mind and it paid off. I wonder how many times we actually remember some data but allow it to be erased by doubt.

Strategies and Successful Use of Them

The above story is about more than just learning names. It gives you a formula which you may use to improve many areas in your life.

- First, find an expert
- Second, find out his or her strategy
- Third, copy the behavior
- Fourth, act as if you are able to do it already

Preferred Seating Arrangement

Many of us are accustomed to rooms which are rectangular and we teach from one end of a vertical orientation. It is much more effective whenever possible to teach from the wide end of the room. It brings the students closer to you in proximity which helps communication. Learning is increased by changing the layout of the room you use regularly in order to keep people alert. People attending safety meetings sometimes have a resistant attitude when it comes to training. By breaking their pattern it is possible to teach more effectively.

The horizontal setup is more effective as the trainees are closer to the speaker. The nearer you are to the people you are addressing the more connected you will be. Distance from a stage to the audience can be overcome by the speaker moving around throughout the audience. This motion also causes the people in the audience to change their physical position which helps keep them alert and breaks their normal pattern of passively watching a speaker.

Changing the layout of the room allows you to break trainees' mental patterns. By breaking their pattern it is possible to teach more effectively.

Treating Trainees As An Audience

You may notice throughout my presentations that I refer to those being trained as the audience. I do this for several reasons. First, I have had many years experience entertaining audiences with storytelling, public speaking and magic. In the past several years I have been blessed with the realization that entertainment can be used to effectively teach. This method has been used throughout time. Jesus taught in parables (stories with a message). With only a three year speaking career He changed history. Parents use many stories to teach their children concepts which may be abstract. The fact is we like hearing stories and while we are entertained, we also learn. Modern writers such as Kenneth Blanchard and Og Mandino use stories to convey business and personal development ideas.

If you accept my premise that teaching or training can be enhanced by entertaining then you understand why I use the term audience. If you want to be an effective trainer you must meet the needs of your audience. They must be comfortable, able to see and hear your message. In order to be effective you must maximize their ability to learn. You must respect their needs.

Public Address Systems

If you let your ego get involved you will make the mistake I made for many years of assuming I was capable of working without a PA system. I failed to realize that for some of my audience I was not able to be heard due to their particular situation and resources. As a result they missed out on some or all of my message, humor or entertainment.

People like and prefer amplification but hate poor public address systems. In many cases the problems with amplification systems can be overcome by a little preparation and practice. If you are in the business of communicating and as a trainer you are, you must become familiar with tools which will enhance communication. I am not going to attempt to give you statistics which show the effectiveness of using amplification. I will; however, share with you my experience based upon 19 years of making presentations before groups. I have been blessed with a booming voice and I learned to speak and entertain groups through the Boy Scouts of America. As a result I learned to project to large audiences even when a PA system wasn't available. For years I would go without a PA because I did not want to be bothered. I honestly believed as you also probably do, that I was being heard by my entire audience. Recently, I began using a PA system at all of my presentations, both training and entertainment. I was shocked by the result. In many instances there were people in the audience who had been on attendance at one of my previous presentations. At every show without exception someone who was familiar with my work came up to me following the show and told me how much more effective I was and that the entire presentation was much more powerful. What a shock! I then began to notice that those people in the back of the room were more alert and responded to my spoken material much more than before.

Even when you are teaching a small group you need amplification. Amplification can overcome distracting noises i.e. air conditioning and people talking to one another which is very common.

PLEASE DON'T WAIT AS LONG AS I DID TO LEARN THE LESSON: ALWAYS USE AN AMPLIFICATION SYSTEM WHEN TRAINING. ALWAYS, YOU ASK? YES, ALWAYS!

How Many People Are Hearing Impaired?

I did a series of employee safety presentations for a power company outside of California and my last presentation was for only two workers. At first I was not going to use my public address system but I decided to be true to my own beliefs and what I teach. At the end of the presentation both of the workers thanked me for the outstanding presentation and left. I then noticed one of them had come back into the room. He approached and thanked me for using the amplification. He informed me he had worked there for over ten years and this was the first training session he had ever heard. You see people with hearing impairments known or unknown have strategies to succeed and hide their condition.

How many of the people you are talking to are having trouble hearing you?

The Magic of Physiology

There is always an emphasis placed on body language when you study modern communication methods. Many of you may even have read a book or two on the subject. What is fascinating to me is that we don't need to read a book because we are already experts at interpreting body language. Think of a time in your life when you watched a couple in a restaurant talking. You could tell without hearing their words or tone of voice if they were having a positive or a negative experience. The body language they were displaying made it clear to you exactly what was going on. Your physiology and tonality can be a potential barrier to your message. According to a study done at UCLA, congruency of communication is: 7% words, 38% tonality, and 55% physiology. This is a fact you have experienced, even if you haven't focused on it. How many of you, in your life's experiences, can recall a situation when someone's physiology told you just how intense they felt or exactly what they meant?

How does this affect you as a safety communicator? First, it reinforces what I said about being passionate about your message and being committed to your outcomes for your students. If you walk into a training session not wanting to be there or feeling yourself that the material you are about to cover is boring it will come across in your physiology. On the plus side when you are congruent and your physiology conveys the same message as your words you have increased the effectiveness of your communication.

Podium Use And Its Negative Effect

Knowing physiology strengthens your message, you now know the reason for the next suggestion I have for trainers. NEVER USE A PODIUM! What do you see many speakers do? They stand behind a podium. When they do this what happens? Suddenly the message they are sending gets blocked. The audience sees less than half of the speaker. In addition, it is common for people, especially if they are uncomfortable in front of a group, to hold on to the podium for security. This adds another problem, it locks up the speakers hands thereby crippling their gestures. The small portion of their body visible to the audience is not conveying the message they intend, instead it is alerting the audience that the speaker is nervous.

Having a small table with water to drink and a place for your notes can be helpful but carry only the notes you need at that moment and stand away from the table. If you must use notes put them in plastic page protectors and number them with a transparent marking pen so if they are dropped you can have someone in the audience put them back in order as you continue. Don't be afraid to use notes but don't read to your audience. If you listen to talk radio you may have noticed that the best hosts do not let anyone read something. It is boring and lacks the passion of your own words. Remember, your outcome is to motivate people to be safe therefore you do not have to be as polished as a TV newscaster because your message will be carried by your voice and the way you carry yourself. You will be amazed how much more effective you will become. You can still gesture while holding a page of notes.

Use Your Notes In A Creative Way

When you are participating in any activity it is easy to get distracted. People in a room will allow their attention to wander looking at whatever is in a room. Why not use this to our advantage? Keeping in mind that it is a good idea to use walls, etc. to tack up our speaking notes it is possible to put these up in the form of posters or slogans which could be placed around the room. When people are distracted by these they will in fact be reading the material you are teaching anyway and it will increase their retention because of the increased repetition. This will also help reach those who learn visually.

Make Some Training Meetings Special

My clients have found that the effectiveness of their safety meetings is improved by occasionally doing something exceptional at a safety meeting. This breaks the routine and keeps their employees looking forward to the next meeting. There are many ways to make a meeting special. Bring in an outside speaker. How about having me come to your training session? Call (800) 588-9419 (Notice the clever, not so subliminal hint?) Serve refreshments, have a safety luncheon or do something you know your employees would enjoy. This is an opportunity to get your employees involved. They can be a part of choosing what special events they would like. When you are walking around your facility ask individuals by name what ideas they have. If they say they don't know respond by saying, "I know you don't know but if you did know what would you want to do?" Take notes and when you use someone's suggestion give them credit.

Taking Out Time For Training

One of my clients was having trouble getting his or her middle managers to take time out for safety training. It struck me as interesting that as humans we allow ourselves the opportunity to learn as children all the way through college but to take time out of work for training is looked upon as impossible. We accept the fact that we must be trained to begin a job but to interrupt that job to get additional training or information is unacceptable. How do we expect ourselves and our employees to improve if we don't allow them the opportunity to grow?

Handouts With Blank Spaces - A Clever Addition

Make handouts that have the outline of your presentation with blanks where certain key points or words would be. As you do your presentation people in the training session can fill in the notes. This allows them to take notes without the stress of writing down complete sentences. In order to make sure they don't leave with an incomplete set of notes give them something special. Make the last page of your handout an answer key showing the page number and the number of blanks with the words listed so they can fill them in if they missed hearing them or if you covered other material and didn't get to some points in your presentation. The handout should have your fundamental ideas to assure yourself that they have the information you have given them.

Taking Breaks

Flexibility is crucial to being effective in your communications. I take breaks based upon how I evaluate the physiology of the audience. Taking a break because a certain amount of time has elapsed is not flexible and could interrupt a moment which is very productive. I will watch my audience for clues that tell me it's time to either take a break or do some fun stretching exercise which will wake them up.

Opportunities For Learning

Use normal everyday events as opportunities for training. When you teach use questions that arise or incidents that occur as jumping off points; therefore, maintaining the flexibility to teach material as it is meaningful during a training session. The more familiar you are with your material the easier this will be. During each day, events occur which allow you to discuss safety with employees. News events, or being alert when someone does something right allows you to make safety training an ongoing activity. During my live presentations if an event occurs which would illustrate a point I am planning on making during the session I immediately teach that idea or concept because it is much more relevant and easier for people to understand. Flexibility to adapt to opportunities that come your way will increase your effectiveness.

Plan Ahead For The Spontaneous

I once had the opportunity to spend an entire day with one of my mentors and I asked him if he had experienced certain repetitive things in his presentations that I had noticed during the past nine years. He said, "Yes, that when you do the same activity over a span of years certain situations occur repeatedly." If you take the time to watch you become aware of situations which would be natural opportunities to teach some of the concepts you want to teach. For example, I always want to make it a point to talk about proper lifting techniques. As a result I always create a situation in my presentation when I drop something apparently by accident but in fact I have planned it. I then ask for someone to pick the item up for me. I observe their lifting technique and then point it out to the class. So, if you think because of past experience that an opportunity will present itself to make a certain point, wait for it to happen, then if it does not, create the situation to teach that concept.

Chapter 12

Effective Implementation

"The outcomes you hold yourself accountable for are the ones you will achieve."

-- John W. Drebinger Jr.

"Writing in a journal not only creates a record of your life and ideas but becomes a doorway to new ideas, decisions and pathways in the future."
-- John W. Drebinger Jr.

Now Is The Time To Take Action!

Well, congratulations for making it to the end. If you are one of those people that check out the endings of books first, Hi! If you read the chapter on how to use this book and took my suggestions then the back pages of this book should be filled with ideas you like enough to write down and also the location in the book in which you found them. Hopefully, you have taken action on most if not all of them, otherwise take a few moments and read them through to see what action needs to be taken next. May I suggest you pick just one action, then write down the first step you need to take toward its implementation. Put the book down now and go for it! I am sure as you use these ideas you will see your communication with others improving.

"The secret of getting ahead is getting started."
-- Sally Berger

Action Is The Key To Success

Possessing all the knowledge needed to accomplish something is useless unless it is put into action. All of these new communication tools are only valuable when you use them. In other words, actions speak louder than words. You have been exposed to many of my words, over thirty two thousand to be exact, but without taking action on what you have learned there is no advantage to having the knowledge. So have some fun playing with the concepts and putting your whole being into becoming the master communicator I know you can be.

An Example of Someone Taking Action

Just sixty days after my most recent Dynamic Safety Meetings Institute, (More information on this at the end of this chapter) I received a letter from one of the graduates as to how he had already put into action that which he had learned. I include it here so you can use it as a model or inspiration for what you might wish to do. It also shows the value of some new information I have available for you.

Letter From a Dynamic Safety Meetings Institute Graduate

"I wanted to give you an update on what has happened since learning with you in Las Vegas. As you know, I live in Denmark so on my return flights I was able to read your book 4 times and filled it with yellow highlights and noted lots of ideas on separate paper. I listened to your tapes 10 times going to and from work. I came back with a passion to make a difference and my safety partner caught the fever after I shared some of the ideas. We have worked hard to put together a meaningful, fun and structured long term safety campaign called, "Handle with Care". Our target audience is our oil and gas production platform operating 120 miles offshore in the North Sea. We thought it was hard work (but very exciting and rewarding). It was essential that we impart the spirit of the campaign to our offshore Safety Reps and Improvement Supervisors to help us COMMUNICATE a consistent and clear message.

I conducted the kick-off meeting for each team along with one of our three highest ranking company officers. The first kick-off was last week and I was quite nervous and although one of my tricks failed (Blaine's heal and reseal coke can) I was able to use your technique of making my apparent failure into a learning lesson and got many laughs as I was willing to be self-deprecating about the incident. The most important part of the kick-off was to get the team to make a statement regarding the possibility of zero injuries. I used the needle through the balloon trick to challenge their beliefs that zero is impossible.

I accomplished that by giving each audience member a small sheet of paper with two questions: How many lost time injuries have occurred on the platform in 2002? How many lost time injuries do you believe we can achieve in 2003? I then asked them to go to the big papers on the wall and write their answers to the question, "Who or what is most important in your life today?" While they were writing on the board I read the previous answers and I learned two things. Most everyone knew that we had three lost time injuries in 2002 and that about half of the audience did not believe that zero lost time injuries was achievable. That was great! Now I had them where I wanted them. I would be able to share the results of the survey with them and encourage them for knowing about our injuries and then inform them that we don't all believe that zero injuries is possible and how important it is that we agree as a team about that. Then I went through the process of finding a volunteer from the audience. My perfect volunteer was a member of the management team and I knew that the team would really enjoy them as the volunteer. I did the routine of getting him PPE such as glasses, ear protection and some gloves. Finally I brought out the balloon. I explained that my volunteer was now properly protected to take this 40 cm needle and put it through the balloon without popping it. It was perfect, as soon as I said "without popping" he jumped back and said "HOW?". It couldn't have been a better opening to talk about beliefs. After the short talk I said that I would do the job since he didn't believe it was possible and I took the needle from him. When I put the needle through the balloon there was great surprise and applause, it really made a lasting impression. I then went to the wall where I had written out some statistics but had it covered so that it was not a distraction. I showed them other companies that have achieved zero injuries for a long period of time. I let them know about several platforms in the North Sea that have achieved more than a year without a lost time injury, one of which belongs to our company in the United

Kingdom. I really think that hitting them with the facts after busting their mental block with the balloon was powerful. I closed up by talking about what they wrote on the wall papers about what was important to them. Then I told them two personal stories to bring the point home.

I closed the meeting and asked them to fill out the "Feedback Form" and explained how important it was for me to get their input. Each and every person filled it out and I was quite scared to read them because about half of these folks had been up for twelve hours and were just finishing their shift and needed to eat, relax and get to sleep before starting back in less than twelve hours. And I was using forty-five minutes of their very limited and precious time. The Offshore Installation Manager commented how they never have a meeting for more than twenty minutes max because it had been impossible to keep the guys attention or keep them from falling asleep. That made me feel better but I still did not know if I succeeded in getting through to them with the message. Then I went to my cabin to read the responses. I was quite shocked! Every person loved the meeting and was surprised that safety could be fun and get meaningful information across! I did not have one negative comment. People were able to explain what they learned (zero is possible) and everyone wanted more meetings like this one and half the folks were interested in helping to plan future safety campaigns. My favorite comment was, "I never knew safety meetings could be held in a stand-up comedian format!"

John, I am indebted to you and know that I will never be the same since listening to you and catching the infection of making a difference when I communicate. I apologize for the length of this note but I felt I had to give you some description for you to fully understand how much you have impacted me."

- **Michael Clowers**

Thanks

At the beginning of this book I wrote a few paragraphs to thank people who have helped me over the years. Now is the time when I get to thank you for your part in this book. Without a reader and people who have asked me to write this information in book form I would have no purpose in this task. I wish to thank you for your investment of time in reading this, which makes my investment in writing it worthwhile. To help you get the most out of it, try doing some of the following exercises to increase your effectiveness in these techniques.

1. Write an action plan for each of the valuable ideas you wrote down. Remember to include the first step that must be taken and begin.
2. Ask yourself the questions from the beginning of each chapter, designed to help you come up with answers from within you and not just from within this text.
3. Read the book again. A friend once pointed out to me that it takes an author many hours to produce a book and to think you can get all there is to get from it in one reading is a very arrogant attitude. Read it again and see how many more new ideas spring to your mind.

There is more!

If you have enjoyed what you have read, I have a favor to ask. Take a moment to read this and the next page so I can tell you about how you can learn even more. For years, many people have asked me for additional material to help them become more effective. In 2001, I developed the Dynamic Safety Meetings Institute. The Institute, a three-day event held each year, focuses on how to make safety meetings fun, effective, interesting, and motivational. As you know, giving people information just isn't enough. If you are missing the motivational element you will not see a change in behavior. From eight in the morning until five in the afternoon, a room full of safety professionals participated in learning and sharing how to be the most effective safety communicators possible. The best news is that all the material we covered is stuff you can do. I have synthesized the best of my and others' techniques and shared everything during this institute. Now, I know it isn't possible for all of you to attend in person (but if it were how would you make it happen?). We have taken care of that for you. A professional sound engineer recorded all I had to say plus we had all audience comments made on a microphone so that you could benefit from the wisdom of others in attendance. I personally edited the three days into 24 CD's totaling over fourteen hours. This, along with all the materials the participants received is now our Dynamic Safety Meetings Home Study Course. I hope you will take a moment to look at the last page of this book and the inside back cover to see what is included in this powerful course. I would love to have you to share live and in person what each attendee experienced. Because of this, I am making the offer that you can apply the entire purchase price of the home study course to the very next year's live Dynamic Safety Meetings Institute. This means that you can learn from the Home Study Course now and when you attend in person it is like you received the Home Study Course for free! Take a moment and go to page 158 and find out how you can get all these benefits now. Or check out our website at: www.drebinger.com

One last thought is that you may encounter people who do not have the wisdom you possess to continually try to improve their ability to communicate. Perhaps you could share with them the following quote.

"When people have trouble communicating, the least they can do is to shut up."
                                                    - Tom Lehrer

Have fun communicating and having an impact on safety in today's workplace.

Collection of
Empowering Quotes

"If you can't annoy somebody, there's little point in writing."
-Kingsley Amis

"Committing your thoughts to print creates a void in your
mind which your creative spirit will fill with new ideas"
- John W. Drebinger Jr.

"Writing down your thoughts is like planting them in fertile
soil." - John W. Drebinger Jr.

"The effectiveness of communication is gauged by the
results." - John W. Drebinger Jr.

"The mere belief that you can do something begins the
process that makes it happen." - John W. Drebinger Jr.

"The only thing scarier than change is being left behind."
                                                    -- Jim Connery.

"Good teaching is one-fourth preparation and three-fourths
theater." - Gail Godwin

"Work is either fun or drudgery. It depends on your
attitude. I like fun." - Colleen C. Barrett

"To effectively communicate, we must realize that we are all
different in the way we perceive the world and use this
understanding as a guide to our communication with
others." - Anthony Robbins

"Employees don't care about what you know about them,
they care about how much you care about them."
- Harvey Mackay

"Rapport is the ability to enter someone else's world, to
make him feel that you understand him, that you have a
strong common bond. It is the essence of successful
communication." - Anthony Robbins

"Enthusiasm is the footprint left by passion!"
- John W. Drebinger Jr.

"Do not wait for leaders; do it alone, person to person."
- Mother Teresa

"Never doubt that a small, group of thoughtful, committed citizens can change the world. Indeed, it is the only thing that ever has."
- Margaret Mead

"I discovered I always have choices and sometimes it's only a choice of attitude." - Judith M. Knowlton

"Aerodynamically the bumblebee shouldn't be able to fly but the bumblebee doesn't know that so it goes on flying anyway." - Mary Kay Ash

"Failure is not an option." - Eugene Kranz

"Training and education without follow up and enforcement is usually ineffective." - Bruce Wilkinson

"Everything works and nothing works. It all depends on the context." - John W. Drebinger Jr.

"Science may have found a cure for most evils, but it has found no remedy for the worst of them all - the apathy of human beings." - Helen Keller

"Ideas, the children of your mind may appear childish or insignificant at first but written down, nurtured and given respect can grow into the revelations of your tomorrow's."
- John W. Drebinger Jr.

"Study as if you were going to live forever; live as if you were going to die tomorrow." - Maria Mitchell

"If you have knowledge, let others light their candles in it."
- Margaret Fuller

"What's in a name? That which we call a rose by any other name would smell as sweet."
- William Shakespeare, Romeo and Juliet

"There are two ways of meeting difficulties. You alter the difficulties or you alter yourself to meet them."
- Phyllis Bottome

"The real voyage of discovery consists not in seeing new landscapes but in having new eyes." - Marcel Proust

"Discover your uniqueness and exploit it in service to others and you are guaranteed success, prosperity and happiness." - Larry Winget

"Whether you think you can or think you can't
- you are right." - Henry Ford

"Everything you do becomes what you make of it."
- John W. Drebinger Jr.

"The outcomes you hold yourself accountable for are the ones you will achieve" - John W. Drebinger Jr.

"Writing in a journal not only creates a record of your life and ideas but becomes a doorway to new ideas, decisions and pathways in the future." - John W. Drebinger Jr.

"The secret of getting ahead is getting started."
- Sally Berger

"When people have trouble communicating, the least they can do is to shut up." - Tom Lehrer

Idea Journal

What Ideas Can I Use To Improve The Safe Behavior Of Myself and Those With Whom I Work?

I believe I can make a difference.

What Ideas Can I Use To Improve The Safe Behavior Of Myself and Those With Whom I Work?

What Ideas Can I Use To Improve The Safe Behavior Of Myself and Those With Whom I Work?

What Ideas Can I Use To Improve The Safe Behavior Of Myself and Those With Whom I Work?

Resources

To develop many of the ideas in this book I have studied and modeled the training styles of several outstanding trainers. A great way to thank those who have helped you in your career and growth is to refer others to them. If you call for information from any of my sources please let them know I gave you their name so they can be aware of my gratitude. For further information you may contact me or the following organizations.

Robbins Research International, Inc.
9191 Towne Centre Drive, Suite 600
San Diego, CA 92122
1 (800) 445-8183

Advanced Neuro Dynamics, Inc.
615 Pi'ikoi St., Suite 1802
Honolulu, Hawaii 96814
Phone: (800) 800-MIND (6463)

American Board of Hypnotherapy
2002 E. McFadden Ave., Suite 100
Santa Ana, CA 92705
Phone: (714) 245-9340

National Speakers Association
1500 South Priest Drive
Tempe, AZ 85281
Phone: (602) 968-2552

American Society of Safety Engineers
1800 East Oakton St.
Des Plaines, Il 60018
Phone: (847) 699-2929

Safety Meeting Presentations
John Drebinger Presentations
13541 Christensen Rd., Suite 200
Galt, CA 95632
Phone: (800) 588-9419 or Phone: (209) 745-9419
Web site: www.drebinger.com
E-Mail: john@drebinger.com

Magic Props & Tricks
Grand Illusions
7704 Fair Oaks Blvd.
Carmichael, CA 95608
Phone: (916) 944-4708
Web site: www.grandillusions.com
E-Mail: magic@grandillusions.com

Luggage & Luggage Repair
Longshore's Luggage
714 J Street
Sacramento, CA 95814
Phone: (916) 443-8757

Speech Coach
Sarah Victory
28200 Hwy 189 N-100
Lake Arrowhead, CA 92352
Phone: (800) 733-8371
Web: www.thevictorycompany.com

Recommended Reading List

Bacon, Jack. <u>My Grandfathers' Clock.</u> ©2001 and
<u>My Stepdaughter's Watch.</u> © 2003 Normandy House,
Houston, TX 77259-1066. ©2001. Phone: 866-447-4622

Blanchard, Ken & O'Connor, Michael. <u>Managing by Values.</u>
Berrett-Koehler. San Francisco, CA ©1997

Canfield, Jack and Hansen, Mark Victor. <u>Chicken Soup
For The Soul.</u> Health Comm. Deerfield Beach, Fl. ©1993.

Carnegie, Dale. <u>How To Win Friends and Influence People.</u>
Simon & Schuster. New York, N.Y. 10020. ©1936.

Cernan, Eugene & Davis, Don. <u>The Last Man on the Moon.</u>
St. Martin's Press. New York, NY. ©1999. 356 pages.

Chaikin, Andrew. <u>A Man On The Moon.</u> Penguin Books.
New York, NY. ©1994. 670 pages.

Geller, E. Scott, <u>The Participation Factor</u>. American Society
of Safety Engineers. IL. ©2002 and <u>Working Safe.</u> Chilton
Book Co. Radnor, PA ©1996 www.safetyperformance.com

Hansen, Mark Victor. <u>The One Minute Millionaire.</u>
Harmony Books. New York, NY. ©2002

<u>The Holy Bible. New International Version.</u> ©1984
International Bible Society. Zondervan Publishing

Hyken, Shep. <u>Moments of Magic</u>. The Alan Press. 11622
Ladue Road, St. Louis, Mo. 63141. ©1993.

James, Tad and Woodsmall, Wyatt. <u>Time Line Therapy</u>.
Meta Publications. Cupertino, Ca. 95015. ©1988.

Johnson, Spencer. Who Moved My Cheese?. G.P. Putnam's Sons. N.Y.,NY ©1998

Krasner, A.M., Ph.D. The Wizard Within. American Board of Hypnotherapy Press. Santa Ana, Ca. 92705. ©1991.

Laborde, Genie Z. Influencing With Integrity. Syntony Publishing. Mountain View, Ca. 94040. ©1987.

LeBlanc, Mark. Growing Your Business!. 1-800-690-0810. ©2000. www.SmallBusinessSuccess.com

Molloy, John T. New Dress for Success. ©1988 and New Women's Dress for Success. Warner Books. New York, NY. ©1988.

Poynter, Dan. The Self Publishing Manual. ©2002 and Is There A Book Inside You? ©1985 Para Publishing. Santa Barbara, CA. ©2002. www.parapublishing.com

Robbins, Anthony. Awaken the Giant Within. Summit Books. New York, N.Y. 10020. ©1991.

Robbins, Anthony. Unlimited Power. Ballantine Books. New York, N.Y. ©1986.

Schwartz, David. The Magic of Thinking Big. Simon & Schuster. N.Y.,NY. ©1959

Thomas, Bob. Walt Disney. Hyperion. N.Y., N.Y. ©1994.

Winget, Larry. How To Write A Book One Page At A Time. Win Publications! Tulsa, OK.. ©1996. www.larrywinget.com

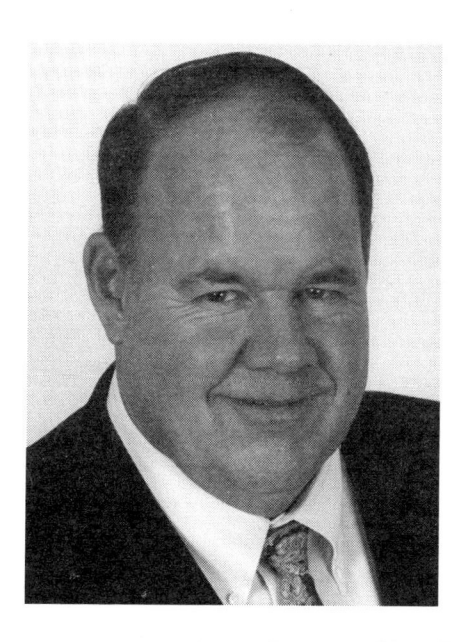

John Warner Drebinger Jr., C.Ht.

John Drebinger works with companies who want a safe workplace and people who want zero injuries. He helps them improve their communication skills. He makes safety fun and interesting. John is considered an expert in safety communication, and in fact has been nicknamed "Master of Safety Communication". He serves a diverse list of clients including, NASA, ExxonMobil, Boeing, Anheuser Busch, IBM, Sony Pictures, and many others. John has a Bachelors Degree in speech and is a Certified Hypnotherapist. John is a member of the National Safety Council and the American Society of Safety Engineers. A member of the National Speakers Association, he has earned their highest earned designation, "Certified Speaking Professional".

To contact: **John Drebinger Presentations**
Toll Free: 1-800-588-9419
Or: 1-209-745-9419
13541 Christensen Rd., Galt, CA, 95632
Email: john@drebinger.com   Web Site: www.drebinger.com

How many lives could you protect... How many dollars could you save... If you knew the secrets of motivation that get results? You want to learn all this and more but can't attend in person...

Now YOU can learn at home, in your car or office!
With John Drebinger's
Dynamic Safety Meetings
Home Study Course

People are dying for passionate, motivational safety meetings!

One of the top motivational safety speakers in the country, **John Drebinger,** is sharing his expertise for creating effective safety meetings. <u>Motivation is the skill of communicating in such a way that causes people to want to take action.</u> Learn the unique secrets he has developed over the years. **When you combine what you know about the content of safety with the techniques John will teach you, the value to your company, your employees , and you is incalculable!**

This groundbreaking program will help you cut injuries by teaching you to:

- Consistently achieve your outcomes;
- Be a resource for solving problems;
- Develop ideas you can use at your next safety meeting;
- Have people look forward to your next safety meeting;
- Be appreciated by employees as a resource who can help;
- Touch the lives of your employees and their families;
- Constantly think of new ways to illustrate a safety concept in a fun way;
- Get compliments from people about your safety meetings;
- Learn to tell safety stories, teaching concepts that people will remember and act upon;
- Learn the secret of writing a safety slogan to communicate your safety message;
- Become aware of methods to determine which Safety Signage is effective and why some are actually harmful;
- Help management discover that safety is an investment that makes money for your company; and,
- See improved safety results.